UNDERSTANDING MENTAL DISORDERS DUE TO MEDICAL CONDITIONS OR SUBSTANCE ABUSE

What Every Therapist Should Know

BRUNNER/MAZEL
BASIC PRINCIPLES INTO PRACTICE SERIES
Series Editor: Natalie H. Gilman

The *Brunner/Mazel Basic Principles Into Practice Series* is designed to present—in a series of concisely written, easily understandable volumes—the basic theory and clinical principles associated with a variety of disciplines and types of therapy. These volumes will serve not only as "refreshers" for practicing therapists, but also as basic texts on the college and graduate level.

1. Family Therapy: Fundamentals of Theory and Practice
   By William A. Griffin, Ph.D.

2. Essentials of Psychoanalysis
   By Herbert S. Strean, D.S.W.

3. Understanding Mental Disorders Due to Medical Conditions or Substance Abuse: What Every Therapist Should Know
   By Ghazi Asaad, M.D.

4. Essentials of Hypnosis
   By Michael D. Yapko, Ph.D.

BRUNNER/MAZEL
BASIC PRINCIPLES INTO PRACTICE SERIES
VOLUME 3

UNDERSTANDING MENTAL DISORDERS DUE TO MEDICAL CONDITIONS OR SUBSTANCE ABUSE

What Every Therapist Should Know

GHAZI ASAAD, M. D.

BRUNNER/MAZEL *Publishers* • NEW YORK

Library of Congress Cataloging-in-Publication Data

Asaad, Ghazi
    Understanding mental disorders due to medical condi-
tions or substance abuse / Ghazi Asaad.
        p.   cm.— (Brunner/Mazel basic principles into
practice series; v.3)
    Includes bibliographical references and index.
    ISBN 0-87630-751-9
    1. Mental illness—Pathophysiology. 2. Psychological
manifestations of general diseases. 3. Mental illness—
Physiological aspects. I. Title. II. Series: Brunner/Mazel
basic principles into practice series; v.3.
    RC455.4.B5A85 1994
    616.89'07—dc20   94-11620
                                                CIP

Published by
BRUNNER/MAZEL, INC.
19 Union Square West
New York, New York 10003

Manufactured in the United States of America
10 9 8 7 6 5 4 3 2 1

To Alia, my wife
with love...

CONTENTS

INTRODUCTION

The purpose of this book is to provide mental health professionals and graduate students with a concise reference on an important category of mental disorders that are caused by general medical conditions, localized brain diseases, or substance abuse. The field of psychotherapy has expanded lately to include many professionals with diverse backgrounds, mostly nonmedical. For that reason, it has become essential to offer all such clinicians a simple access to this complex subject, which represents the interface between Medicine and Psychiatry.

It is particularly important for all clinicians who work with psychiatric patients to become familiar with various mental disorders that are caused by various medical illnesses or substance abuse, since many of these conditions could mimic what are known as "functional" psychiatric disorders. Early recognition and treatment of such mental disorders can be of crucial importance since many serious and potentially fatal medical illnesses may present initially with psychiatric manifestations before the onset of any physical signs or symptoms. Examples include brain tumors, central nervous system infections, and endocrine disorders. This book is intended to facilitate the recognition of psychiatric manifestations of medical conditions and, hence, prompt the clinician to make appropriate medical referrals in a timely fashion.

In this book, I have attempted to avoid medical jargon as much as possible in order to make the material widely accessible. Clinicians and graduate students of various Psychology and Social work Programs will find the book easy to understand and apply in day-to-day clinical practice. It is particularly useful in helping nonmedical psychotherapists understand the nature of mental disor-

Understanding Mental Disorders

ders arising from various medical conditions without their having to review large volumes of medical textbooks and references. However, due to the nature of the subject and in order to preserve scientific accuracy and comprehensiveness, some medical terms and names of medications have been included. Whenever possible, I have attempted to explain those terms in simple language as well.

The subjects discussed in this book were known as "Organic Mental Disorders" until the introduction of DSM-IV (APA, 1994), which eliminated the term "organic." The authors of the DSM-IV, along with many other authors and researchers, felt that the term "organic" might have implied that other psychiatric disorders known as "functional" were somehow unrelated to biological factors. On the contrary, current evidence suggests that all psychiatric disorders, including those labeled as "functional," may be caused by physical factors as well. For example, schizophrenia and panic disorders have been linked to specific neurochemical abnormalities in the brain that can be described as "organic" in nature, although the exact etiology is still unknown. In fact, recent research has shown that physical disorders that cause psychiatric symptoms do so by altering the neurochemistry within the brain in a fashion similar to that occurring in "functional" disorders.

Therefore, it is appropriate to state that psychiatric symptoms arising from both "organic" and "functional" disorders can be caused by abnormalities involving various neurotransmitter systems. Such abnormalities may be induced by known physical factors, as in the cases of strokes and degenerative brain diseases, or by unknown, yet to be confirmed, physical factors, as in the cases of schizophrenia and panic disorders.

The balance between biological and genetic vulnerability on one hand and environmental stressors, physical or psychological, on the other is always crucial in the final equation regarding the manifestation of any given disease, "organic" or "functional." In order to understand this point further, we can examine the example of drug-induced mental disorders. It is widely known that different individuals react differently to the same drug. Under the influence of cocaine, for example, some people experience only elation and increased energy, while others develop paranoid delusions and hallucinations. The difference in patients' responsiveness here is probably due to differences in biological vulnerabilities dictated by genetic factors and by the neurochemistry of the central nervous system in each individual. Similarly, individuals with biological vulnerability towards psychosis or mood disorders may appear to be stable under normal conditions, yet may decompensate and exhibit psychotic or mood changes when subjected to severe environmental stressors of a physical or psychological nature. Using this framework of thinking makes the distinction between "organic" mental disorders and "functional" mental disorders less noticeable. DSM-IV refers to all mental disorders that are not caused by general medical conditions or by substance abuse as "Primary Mental Disorders."

The first chapter in this book presents a historical background on the subject and reviews the definitions and phenomenology of various "organic" conditions. It also discusses brain lesions and their diverse clinical manifestations. The following five chapters discuss various disorders, including dementia, delirium, delusional disorders, hallucinosis, mood disorders, anxiety disorders, and personality change arising from medical conditions. Clinical vignettes are presented to illustrate various conditions and point out diagnostic similarities between "organic" and "primary" psychiatric disorders. The remaining 11 chapters of the book deal with specific "organic" mental disorders, ranging from Alzheimer's disease to drug-induced mental disorders.

The reader will notice that I have attempted repeatedly to make the point that mental disorders arising from medical conditions or substance abuse can be mistaken for "primary" or "functional" disorders. My main goal is to heighten the awareness of all mental health professionals and, especially, students toward physical factors so they can recognize different psychiatric conditions that may be caused by medical illnesses more readily in the course of their work with psychiatric patients in various clinical settings. I hope that by writing *Understanding Mental Disorders Due to Medical Conditions or Substance Abuse,* I have succeeded in this important mission.

1

HISTORY, DEFINITIONS, AND PHENOMENOLOGY

HISTORY

Since the beginning of Medicine, there has been the belief that certain mental disorders are caused by physical factors. Early medical writings described delirium, which was referred to as phrenitis at that time, with great clarity and consistency. In the 4th century B.C., Hippocrates wrote of phrenitis or delirium and defined the condition as a mental disorder associated with physical diseases, especially those of febrile nature.

In the first century, Celsus coined the two famous terms "Delirium" and "Dementia." He designated the term delirium to describe acute mental disorders associated with fevers and elaborated that certain cases of delirium could be followed by dementia continua or true insanity.

Most writers during the 1st and 2nd centuries made a clear distinction between delirium and dementia based on the chronicity of the condition. It was known then that delirium can arise not only from fever but also from drunkenness and poisoning from certain drugs. Galen taught that acute mental illness can arise either from primary cerebral disease or from secondary brain disease in reaction to distant diseased organs, as in the case of pneumonia. Soranus described several cases of delirium and noted that patients with delirium could be hyperac-

1

tive or hypoactive, and may suffer from severe insomnia. In the centuries that followed, several new terms were introduced to describe various forms of "organic" mental disorders. However, the terms delirium and dementia have survived nearly 2000 years, despite inconsistent usage from time to time (Lipowski, 1980a).

Following the fall of Roman civilization, little was added to the concept of "organic" mental disorders. In the 13th century, Thomas Aquinas believed that insanity was primarily a somatic disturbance. He was considered by some psychiatric historians to be the precursor of the so-called organicistic school of psychiatry that became prevalent during the second half of the 19th century in Germany (Mora, 1980). In the 14th, 15th and 16th centuries, knowledge about causes, clinical manifestations, and treatments of delirium and dementia was advanced by several other investigators.

The distinction between delirium and dementia continued to evolve during the 17th century, shedding more light on causes and clinical manifestations. Thomas Willis devoted a book to mental disorders, which he viewed as diseases of the brain. He described both acute and chronic "organic" mental disorders in great detail. Morton, a contemporary of Willis, added that delirium represented a waking dream. That notion was further developed in the 18th century by Quincy, who elaborated that delirium represented dreams of waking persons with excited incoherent ideas and irregular fluctuations. These views in relation to pathophysiology of delirium remain valid to the present date (Lipowski, 1980a).

The 19th century witnessed significant advances in medical knowledge. The concept of "organic" mental disorders was further refined and integrated to highlight the correlation between physical illness and mental disorders. Pinel and Esquirol made significant contributions towards the progress of the understanding of "organic" mental disorders. Others, with equally important contributions to the field, included Rush, Prichard, and Griesinger (Zilboorg, 1941).

The contributions of Bonhoeffer towards acute "organic" mental disorders had far-reaching effects on the progress of organic psychiatry in the beginning of the 20th century. This was followed by equally important work conducted by Bleuler, who focused his attention on chronic "organic" mental disorders and made invaluable contributions to the field (Lipowski, 1980a).

The second half of the 20th century has witnessed remarkable progress in the field of mental disorders due to medical conditions. This was largely due to technological advances in the areas of brain imaging, including computerized axial tomography (CAT) scan, magnetic resonance imaging (MRI), positron emission tomography (PET), and single photon emission computed tomography (SPECT) scans. In addition, brain research focusing on molecular neurobiology and neurotransmitters has exploded over the past decade and contributed immensely to our current understanding of brain functions and mental illness (Yudofsky & Hales, 1992).

DEFINITIONS

"ORGANIC" MENTAL DISORDERS refer to a group of psychiatric disorders caused by permanent damage to or temporary dysfunction of the brain (Lipowski, 1980b). The underlying cerebral disease may be primary in nature, involving anatomical, neurophysiological, or biochemical changes arising within the brain tissue itself, or it may be secondary to a systemic disease involving other organs.

Examples of mental disorders that are caused by primary brain diseases include delirium in association with head injury, hallucinations occurring in temporal lobe epilepsy, and dementia resulting from Parkinson's disease. Examples of secondary mental disorders include delirium in association with hepatic failure, anxiety in the course of thyroid disease, and dementia associated with anemia and vitamin B12 deficiency. Other examples of secondary mental disorders include intoxications with alcohol, drugs, and various pharmacological agents.

The term "organic" has served the purpose of distinguishing mental disorders that are caused by physical factors from those that were presumed to be "functional" in nature. However, current evidence strongly suggests that all mental disorders are probably caused by "organic" factors. For this reason, the most recent edition of the *Diagnostic and Statistical Manual of Mental Disorders* (DSM-IV, 1994) has eliminated the term "organic" completely and classified all "organic" mental disorders under delirium, dementia, amnestic disorders, mental disorders due to a general medical condition, and substance-related disorders. Furthermore, DSM-IV (1994) uses the term "primary" mental disorders to refer to all other mental disorders including those known as "functional" mental disorders.

DELIRIUM refers to an acute mental disorder characterized by disturbances in cognition and in the ability to maintain attention to external stimuli. The patient is often disoriented, agitated, and incoherent, and may experience various forms of hallucinations and illusions. Occasionally, the level of consciousness is reduced; sometimes, the patient is unable to remain awake during the examination. The disorder is typically of a transient duration, the length of which depends on the underlying etiology. Delirium can be caused by a wide variety of medical conditions. Examples include uremia and intoxication with anticholinergic medications.

DEMENTIA refers to a chronic mental disorder characterized by impairment of memory and intellect, and by personality changes. Typically, the level of consciousness is not affected. The onset is insidious and the course is often progressive. Like delirium, dementia can be caused by a wide variety of medical conditions. Examples include Alzheimer's disease and AIDS dementia.

AMNESTIC DISORDER is a term used in DSM-IV (1994) to refer to impairment in short- and long term memory that is caused by specific factors. Examples include amnestic disorders associated with alcoholism and thiamine deficiency.

CONFUSION is a term often used by clinicians to describe a variety of conditions. It generally refers to symptoms and signs that indicate that the patient is unable to think with his or her customary clarity and coherence (Lishman, 1987). It is often used to describe disorientation in cases of delirium, dementia, or psychosis. This term has limited usefulness due to its lack of specificity. For that reason, the use of the term should be avoided unless further clinical description is provided.

HALLUCINOSIS refers to hallucinatory symptoms of various forms that occur in clear states of consciousness in the absence of other psychotic symptoms such as delusions or thought disorder. The condition is caused by specific physical factors and can be persistent or recurrent. Examples include prolonged use of alcohol and temporal lobe epilepsy (Asaad, 1990).

MOOD DISORDER DUE TO MEDICAL CONDITIONS refers to either a depressive or elated state that can arise as a result of physical disorders. Examples include thyroid disease and side effects to corticosteroids.

ANXIETY DISORDER DUE TO MEDICAL CONDITIONS denotes prominent and recurrent panic attacks or anxiety symptoms that are caused by certain illnesses. Examples include hypoglycemia and pulmonary embolism.

PERSONALITY CHANGE DUE TO MEDICAL CONDITIONS refers to persistent disturbance in behavior characterized by recurrent outbursts of rage, impaired social judgment, and affective instability. Frontal lobe tumors and temporal lobe epilepsy are leading examples of this condition.

PHENOMENOLOGY

Mental disorders due to medical conditions or substance abuse usually manifest with cognitive, emotional, and behavioral symptoms, depending on the nature of the underlying disease, the areas involved, and the severity of the illness. The clinical presentation of each disorder may vary considerably, and is usually heavily influenced by the patient's premorbid personality organization, intellectual and educational level, and psychodynamic background (Lishman, 1987).

The types of physical factors that can cause temporary dysfunction or permanent damage to the brain involve a great number of pathological processes. Head injury, brain tumors, strokes, autoimmune diseases, degenerative brain diseases, metabolic disorders, and infections are examples of such processes.

LEVEL OF CONSCIOUSNESS changes often occur in reaction to an acute disorder such as head trauma or intoxication. The degree of impairment of consciousness can vary depending on the type and degree of injury, the areas of the brain affected, and the age and physical condition of the patient. Older individuals, especially those who are physically debilitated, are at a greater risk for developing alterations in their level of consciousness. Furthermore, in the same individual, the level of consciousness can fluctuate from time to time within the same day. For instance, delirious patients tend to suffer from further impairment in their consciousness towards nighttime. Impairment in consciousness can vary from mild inattentiveness to the environment to severe impairment of consciousness to the degree of coma. In between the two extremes, variable degrees of impairment can be encountered. Often, the sleep-wakefulness cycle is disrupted, and most patients report insomnia and vivid dreams (Lipowski, 1980b).

BEHAVIORAL CHANGES develop in the course of mental disorders due to medical conditions or substance abuse. In acute conditions, such as delirium, the patient is often agitated and highly irritable, although in some instances the patient may become subdued and unresponsive. Increased psychomotor activity in cases of acute disorders is often characterized by being purposeless and automatic. Startle reactions are common. Combative and assaultive behavior can develop. In chronic disorders, such as dementia, on the other hand, behavioral changes often are subtle and insidious. Typically, the patient begins to show signs of disinhibition such as making inappropriate remarks or exhibiting inappropriate sexual behavior. Usually, the patient shows little affect concerning his or her inappropriate behavior. Occasionally, the patient may become angry or agitated.

HALLUCINATIONS AND ILLUSIONS are common in cases of acute disorders. Typically, visual hallucinations are more common than others, and simple unformed types of hallucinations are more frequent than complex ones. However, tactile, auditory, olfactory, and gustatory hallucinations occur frequently. In addition, highly formed complex hallucinations are not uncommon. Hallucinations of similar nature can also occur in cases of chronic disorders (Asaad, 1990).

DISORIENTATION for time, place, and person can occur in both acute and chronic disorders. Disorientation is usually profound in cases of acute disorders, although in advanced cases of chronic disorders equally profound disorientation may be observed. In both situations, disorientation for time develops early and is later followed by disorientation for place, and then for person.

MEMORY IMPAIRMENT is a cardinal symptom in dementias and other amnestic disorders. The onset is usually gradual and involves recent memory. Long-term memory is usually preserved until the final stages of the disease. Typically, the patient is unaware of his or her memory difficulties, and tends to confabulate. Memory impairment also occurs in the course of acute disorders. However, this impairment is transient and is largely due to difficulties in paying attention to the environment, perceiving the stimulations, and comprehending the information.

THINKING DISTURBANCES can be encountered in the course of acute disorders. The patient may not be able to think coherently or logically. Reality testing may become impaired and the patient may express bizarre ideas and fantasies. Ideas of reference and paranoid delusions can occur. In chronic disorders, the thinking process is generally slow and impoverished. Abstract thinking is usually lost, along with the ability to reason and plan. Intellectual capacity is diminished over time; in most patients, insight and judgment are compromised.

SPEECH can be affected in mental disorders due to medical conditions or substance abuse. In acute conditions, the patient's speech is often incoherent, loud, and repetitive. In chronic conditions, disturbance in speech is progressive and tends to mirror the underlying thinking process.

MOOD CHANGES AND ANXIETY occur in mental disorders due to medical conditions or substance abuse. Depressive or manic symptoms can develop in acute as well as chronic disorders. Associated features including sleep and appetite disturbances as well as suicidal ideation, and attempts at suicide can occur. Severe anxiety and panic attacks in the course of mental disorders due to medical conditions or substance abuse may resemble to a large extent primary anxiety and panic disorders, respectively.

CLINICAL MANIFESTATIONS OF BRAIN LESIONS

As indicated earlier, the signs and symptoms encountered in the course of any mental disorder resulting from medical conditions or substance abuse depend, at least in part, on the areas of the brain that are involved in the injury or the dysfunction. This observation is of special importance since it may alert the physician to the nature and extent of the underlying illness, and prompt the initiation of appropriate diagnostic tests and specific treatment. It is important to emphasize here that, in addition to psychiatric symptoms, various physical and, especially, neurological signs and symptoms are likely to be present.

FRONTAL LOBE lesions typically produce symptoms of behavior changes consisting of social disinhibition and poor judgment. Inappropriate sexual behavior and general indifference to serious situations often occur. The patient seldom shows signs of anxiety or any other meaningful emotional responses; instead, he or she may show elevated mood with empty affect. Emotional lability with rapid shifts between tearfulness and euphoria may be observed. Cognitive functions, including concentration, calculation, abstract thinking, and planning ability may become compromised.

In addition, several neurological signs and symptoms may develop, including motor weakness or paralysis, gait disturbances, exaggerated reflexes, and the emergence of the grasp reflex as well as a positive Babinski response. Disturbances in language functions may occur if the lesion involves the dominant hemisphere. Visual abnormalities can occur due to orbital lesions. Urinary as well as fecal incontinence may occur relatively early in the course of the illness (Lishman, 1987).

PARIETAL LOBE lesions generally do not produce specific psychiatric symptoms. Common neurological signs and symptoms include sensory impairment, spatial disorientation, language disturbances, agraphia, and visual abnormalities (Peele, 1977).

TEMPORAL LOBE lesions may lead to a variety of psychiatric symptoms. Most commonly, personality changes similar to those observed in frontal lobe lesions develop. Aggressive outbursts and emotional instability can occur. Other symptoms include various forms of hallucinations and psychotic symptoms, depression, anxiety, cognitive impairment, and changes in the level of consciousness. Automatism and other seizure-related phenomena are common (Gastaut & Broughton, 1972). Neurological signs and symptoms of temporal lobe lesions include language impairment, memory disturbances, visual field defects, and epilepsy.

OCCIPITAL LOBE lesions produce mainly visual hallucinations and illusions (Asaad, 1990). Other visual abnormalities, including visual field defects, are common.

2

DELIRIUM

DEFINITION AND CLINICAL FEATURES

Lipowski (1980a) defines delirium as "a transient organic mental disorder characterized by the global impairment of cognitive functions, acute onset, and widespread disturbance of cerebral metabolism." Typically, the patient shows reduced ability to maintain attention to external stimuli, with variable degrees of alteration in the level of consciousness. Arousal is either reduced or heightened, and often there is disturbance in the sleep-wakefulness cycle. The patient may be consistently or intermittently drowsy during the daytime and may display insomnia at night. Psychomotor activity may be increased or decreased, with rapid shifts between the two states.

Cognitive impairment involves disturbances in concentration, recent memory, registration, thinking, and orientation. Disorientation for time is most common, wherein the patient is unable to state the date, the day of the week, and the time of day correctly. Disorientation for place occurs less often, and refers to the patient's inability to identify his or her surroundings and location correctly. For example, a patient in a hospital may think that he or she is at work. Disorientation for person may develop in severe cases of delirium wherein the patient is unable to identify people correctly. The patient may mistake a nurse at the hospital for his wife.

The patient's ability to think coherently is reduced, and thinking becomes disorganized, slowed, or accelerated. Often, the patient is unable to reason or problem-solve. Paranoid delusions of transient and poorly systematized nature may occur. Memory disturbances involve inability to register new information and impairment of recent recall of events that occurred before the onset of delirium (Lipowski, 1980b).

Perceptual disturbances are particularly common in delirium. Visual and auditory illusions are frequent. For example, the patient may perceive cracks in the wall as snakes crawling, or may perceive the sound of footsteps as someone banging on the door. Hallucinations are mostly of the visual type. Patients experience seeing simple images consisting of circles, lines, geometric figures, and flashes of colors and light. Frequently, they report seeing insects and small animals. Occasionally, frightening images develop which may force the patient to flee and, consequently, injure himself or others in the process. Simple as well as complex auditory, tactile, olfactory, and gustatory hallucinations occur in delirium as well (Asaad, 1990).

The onset is usually rapid and the course is transient. Depending on the underlying medical condition, the duration may last from a few hours to several days. Rarely, it may last for weeks or longer. Delirium is often intermittent and tends to fluctuate over the course of a day. Typically, the symptoms are worse in the evening and at nighttime. Patients may display lucid intervals, with normal mental status examination during daytime.

Associated features include fear and anxiety, depression, irritability, euphoria, and apathy. In addition, several physical and neurological signs and symptoms are observed, depending on the underlying etiology. Common findings include elevated temperature, elevated blood pressure, tachycardia, sweating, and abnormal laboratory findings.

ETIOLOGY AND PATHOPHYSIOLOGY

Delirium can be produced by a wide variety of medical conditions, some of which arise within the brain itself, while others arise in distant organs and adversely affect brain functions. Pathological processes that can contribute to deliria include traumatic brain injuries, intracerebral bleeding, brain tumors, intracranial infection, systemic infection, acute renal failure, acute hepatic failure, endocrine disturbances, drug and chemical intoxication, alcohol and drug withdrawal, and others. A comprehensive list is provided in Table 1.

Older patients, especially those over 75 years of age, are more susceptible to delirium. In addition, patients with debilitating illness, preexisting brain damage, or a history of alcohol or drug abuse are at higher risk (Lipowski, 1980b).

The exact mechanism of pathophysiology of delirium is not fully known. It has been suggested that the basic etiology of delirium is a dysfunction in the metabolism of the brain. EEG tracings often show generalized slowing, and occasionally show low-voltage fast activity. EEG changes seem to correlate significantly with clinical presentation, and are thought to reflect the underlying metabolic abnormalities. Other theories refer to cerebral blood flow changes and brain damage as being implicated in the pathophysiologic process of delirium (Wise & Brandt, 1992).

DIFFERENTIAL DIAGNOSIS AND DIAGNOSTIC CRITERIA

Early detection of delirium is of prime importance, since it usually signifies a serious medical illness that requires immediate attention and treatment. Complete physical examination and appropriate laboratory investi-

---

TABLE 1
CAUSES OF DELIRIUM

A. DISORDERS ARISING WITHIN THE BRAIN:
    1. Head injury
    2. Intracranial hemorrhages
    3. Intracranial tumors
    4. Intracranial infections
    5. Cerebral autoimmune diseases
    6. Seizures

B. DISORDERS ARISING IN DISTANT ORGANS:
    1. Acute renal failure
    2. Acute hepatic failure
    3. Acute cardiac failure
    4. Acute respiratory failure
    5. Systemic infections
    6. Endocrine disturbances
    7. Fluid and electrolyte imbalance

C. INTOXICATIONS:
    1. Pharmacological agents
    2. Alcohol and drugs
    3. Industrial poisons

D. ALCOHOL AND DRUG WITHDRAWAL.

E. MISCELLANEOUS:
    1. Vitamin deficiency and anemia
    2. Hyperthermia or hypothermia
    3. Sensory deprivation and postoperative states
    4. Hypersensitivity and allergic reactions

---

gations are essential. Specific investigations as dictated by the clinical condition, including EEG, must be pursued when indicated. While physical signs and symptoms and laboratory investigations may vary depending on the underlying medical condition, mental status examination is usually consistent and shows signs of alteration in the level of consciousness, disorientation, thinking disorder, hallucinations and illusions, and increased or decreased psychomotor activity. Sudden onset and fluctuation of symptoms are highly characteristic.

Delirium needs to be distinguished from dementia. In dementia, the onset is insidious, the duration is chronic, there is no alteration in the level of consciousness, and the sleep-wakefulness cycle is usually normal for age. Other mental disorders due to medical conditions or substance abuse are distinguished from delirium by the absence of disturbance of consciousness. Psychotic disorders and mood disorders may be difficult to differentiate from delirium in certain cases. EEG is often normal in those conditions. Finally, delirium should be distinguished from factitious and dissociative disorders. In these conditions, mental status examination of cognitive functions shows glaring inconsistencies (Lipowski, 1980b).

Minimental status examination (Folstein, Folstein & McHugh, 1975) is often adequate to elicit essential symptoms. This test takes between 5 and 10 minutes to administer and consists of two sections: the first section covers orientation, memory, and attention; the second section tests the patient's ability to name common objects, follow verbal and written commands, write a sentence spontaneously, and copy a simple figure. Full score is 30, and scores of less than 24 usually indicate cognitive impairment (Lishman, 1987).

Diagnostic criteria for delirium adapted from DSM-IV (1994) are outlined in Table 2.

TABLE 2
DIAGNOSTIC CRITERIA FOR DELIRIUM
(Adapted from DSM-IV, 1994)

A. Disturbance of consciousness with reduced clarity of awareness of the environment and reduced ability to maintain attention to external stimuli.

B. Disturbance of thinking, speech, memory, and orientation, or the onset of perceptual abnormalities such as illusions or hallucinations.

C. The onset is usually acute (hours to days), and the symptoms often fluctuate over the course of the day.

D. The condition is caused by an underlying medical illness, substance intoxication or withdrawl, or medication side effects.

TREATMENT AND PROGNOSIS

Treatment of delirium must be directed at the underlying medical illness that is responsible for the condition. Specific measures should be taken whenever possible. For example; treatment of delirium resulting from anticholinergic intoxication is best achieved by administering a cholinergic agent such as physostigmine to counteract the effects of the toxic drug; and treatment of alcohol withdrawal delirium (delirium tremens) is best achieved by using a benzodiazepine such as Librium along with Thiamine. Treatment of specific medical conditions that can induce mental disorders will be discussed in corresponding chapters.

In addition, general measures can be taken to correct changes in mental status regardless of the underlying medical illness.

1. Environmental Interventions

Delirious patients generally require admission to the hospital for observation and treatment. Frequently, cases of delirium arise in nursing homes where management can be carried out adequately. Patients should be kept in a quiet, well lighted room, preferably with a familiar relative or a staff member present at all times to frequently orient the patient and prevent him or her from accidentally injuring self or others. It has been reported that some patients had jumped out of their hospital room window during delirious states. Many patients attempt to remove tubes and intravenous lines that are essential for their treatment. Physical restraints may be used when necessary. A calendar with big letters and a clock should be placed in the room to keep the patient oriented to time. Placing familiar objects in the room can help the patient remain oriented to the environment.

2. Pharmacological Interventions

Tranquilizers are useful and are often essential for the treatment of delirium. Agitated patients, especially those with hallucinations and paranoid ideation, require such an intervention. Small doses of a high-potency antipsychotic agent such as haloperidol are usually very effective in controlling most of the symptoms of delirium. Low-potency antipsychotic agents should be avoided due to their hypotensive and anticholinergic properties which can exacerbate delirium. Benzodiazepines such as Librium and Lorazepam are effective in cases of delirium that are caused by withdrawel from alcohol and sedatives or by intoxication with cocaine, PCP, and hallucinogens. They can also be used in some patients for sleep induction. However, in certain types of deliria, they can increase the degree of disorientation and disinhibition. Therefore, they should be used with caution (Wise & Brandt, 1992).

3. Supportive Interventions

Patients' vital signs should be monitored regularly and any significant changes need to be addressed appropriately. Adequate hydration and nutrition and correction of electrolyte imbalance are important. Patients often require intravenous infusion of fluids with glucose and saline. Oxygen may be needed in certain patients. General nursing care is provided and may be geared towards specific medical illnesses.

Most delirious patients recover completely, especially when the underlying medical illness is diagnosed and treated effectively. Early diagnosis and treatment are important factors in determining the rate and the degree of recovery. Elderly patients tend to have less favorable outcome and higher mortality rate than younger patients (Liston, 1984). Untreated or inadequately treated cases of delirium may lead to dementia or personality change.

3

DEMENTIA AND AMNESTIC DISORDER

I: DEMENTIA

Definition and Clinical Features

Dementia can be defined as a mental disorder characterized by global impairment in memory and other cognitive functions in a clear state of consciousness. During early stages of dementia, short-term memory deteriorates gradually, along with the ability to learn new information. The patient may forget appointments, telephone numbers, or names. As the dementia progresses, he or she may not be able to remember names of close relatives or even one's own name. Long-term memory remains intact in early stages of dementia. The patient may be able to recall events that took place during childhood, yet fails to remember what he or she ate for breakfast. Eventually, long-term memory is affected and the patient is unable to recall any past event.

Abstract thinking is lost, along with the ability to form concepts, problem-solve, or calculate. Thinking becomes impoverished and the patient is unable to plan or exercise good judgment. Consequently, the patient begins to exhibit signs of social and occupational impairment. For example, a successful businessman may begin to make bad business decisions; or an otherwise shy woman may begin to make inappropriate sexual advances towards her co-workers.

Personality changes develop gradually, and are often detected by family members and friends. The patient becomes forgetful and often misplaces or loses belongings. Dangerous accidents can occur in relation to forgetting to turn off the stove or to smoking in bed. Typically, the patient confabulates in order to compensate for the cognitive deficits. He or she tends to be circumstantial and talk excessively about irrelevant issues and fail to respond to the question directly.

In the early stages of dementia, the patient may become aware of his or her impairment, and may react with anxiety, depression, or withdrawal. As the illness progresses, the patient shows little or no concern regarding his or her cognitive impairment, and continues to pretend and carry out a seemingly normal conversation with other people.

The patient is always alert, yet is often disoriented. Disorientation to time occurs first. The patient may not know the date or the day of the week. The degree of disorientation to time may vary depending on the severity and the nature of the underlying illness that is causing the dementia. Disorientation to place follows, while disorientation to person is delayed until advanced stages of dementia.

In addition, the patient may show signs of impulsivity, emotional lability, and agitation. Other symptoms include violent behavior, suicidal tendencies, delusional thinking, hallucinations and tendency to wander away from home and get lost despite being in familiar surroundings. The patient may accuse family members of stealing his or her belongings. Some patients develop delusions of jealousy towards the spouse and may become violent as a result of their suspicions.

Although dementia occurs more often in the elderly, as in the cases of Alzheimer's disease and vascular dementia, it can occur at any age depending on the underlying causative illness. Dementia in children can be produced by metabolic disorders such as Wilson's disease or by infections such as untreated encephalitis. Dementia in children is often associated with mental retardation and various learning disabilities. The child usually exhibits withdrawal, irritability, and deterioration in school performance.

The onset of dementia is usually insidious except in cases that are preceded by untreated acute "organic" mental disorders. In some cases of dementia where the underlying etiology can be identified and treated early in the process, complete reversal of the symptoms can occur, as in cases of dementia resulting from vitamin deficiency. Untreated or untreatable dementias usually have a progressive course, with gradual deterioration of memory and other intellectual abilities. In early stages, the patient may not show significant signs of impairment, and may be able to cover up or compensate for his or her deficits. Later, the signs and symptoms become obvious even to strangers. In the final stages of the disease, the patient may become totally dependent on others to meet daily needs. Towards the end, the patient may lose the ability to move or speak and may lose control of bladder and bowel functions. Death is usually due to medical complications such as infections and failure of various body organs.

Etiology and Pathophysiology

As in delirium, dementia can be caused by a wide variety of pathological processes that involve the brain directly or indirectly. Conditions that can cause dementia include degenerative brain diseases such as Alzheimer's disease and Parkinson's disease, alcohol abuse leading to Wernicke's encephalopathy and Korsakoff's syndrome, metabolic disorders such as chronic hepatic and renal failure, vascular disorders such as vascular dementia, chronic infections such as tertiary syphilis and AIDS,

---

TABLE 3
CAUSES OF DEMENTIA

A. DEGENERATIVE BRAIN DISEASES:
1. Alzheimer's disease
2. Pick's disease
3. Senile dementia
4. Parkinson's disease
5. Huntington's chorea

B. VASCULAR DISEASES:
1. Vascular dementia/Strokes
2. Subdural hematoma
3. Carotid artery and other arterial occlusion

C. CHRONIC INFECTIONS:
1. AIDS dementia
2. Tertiary syphilis
3. Meningitis
4. Encephalitis
5. Creutzfeldt-Jakob disease

D. METABOLIC DISORDERS:
1. Chronic renal failure
2. Chronic hepatic failure
3. Chronic respiratory and cardiac failure
4. Chronic electrolyte imbalance
5. Wilson's disease
6. Porphyria

E. ENDOCRINE DISORDERS:
1. Hypothyroidism
2. Parathyroid diseases
3. Addison's disease
4. Cushing's syndrome

F. VITAMIN DEFICIENCY:
    1. Folate deficiency
    2. Thiamine deficiency
    3. Vitamin B12 deficiency
    4. Iron deficiency and severe anemia

G. INTOXICATIONS:
    1. Chronic alcohol abuse (Korsakoff's syndrome)
    2. Chronic drug abuse
    3. Heavy metals (lead, mercury, arsenic)

H. MISCELLANEOUS:
    1. Normal pressure hydrocephalus
    2. Space-occupying lesions
    3. Multiple sclerosis
    4. Systemic lupus erythematosus

---

chronic intoxications with heavy metals, and vitamin deficiencies. A comprehensive list is provided in Table 3. Alzheimer's disease is discussed in Chapter Seven. Vascular dementia is discussed in Chapter Eight.

The primary pathological finding in cases of dementia is the widespread involvement of cortical areas with various lesions such as degeneration, infarction, fibrosis, infection, anoxia, or chronic pressure. Damage to subcortical areas of the brain can also be responsible for certain types of dementia (Wells, 1985). The clinical manifestations depend primarily on the areas involved in the pathological process. Most symptoms of dementia arise from lesions in the frontal lobe cortex. Other symptoms arise due to temporal or parietal cortical areas. Specific symptoms that are caused by lesions in certain cortical areas are discussed in Chapter One.

In addition to cerebral pathology, it has been noted that psychosocial factors can influence the onset of dementia as well as its severity and degree of compensation. Premorbid personality organization, degree of intelligence, level of education, and social support systems are of prime importance.

Differential Diagnosis and Diagnostic Criteria

Early diagnosis and treatment of dementia may be of critical value in determining the prognosis. Since dementia is always caused by an underlying medical condition, it is essential to obtain a complete physical examination with appropriate laboratory investigations as indicated. CT scan of the brain is often needed to confirm or rule out certain neurological conditions. Physical signs and symptoms may or may not be present. Mental status examination is essential and reveals significant memory deficit and impairment of most cognitive functions. As a rule, the level of consciousness is not altered, and the patient is not aware of the degree of his or her impairment. Most patients tend to confabulate and to be circumstantial. The onset is often insidious, or may follow an acute mental disorder such as delirium.

Dementia should be differentiated from delirium, pseudodementia, normal aging, and amnestic disorder. In delirium, the onset is acute and the level of consciousness often fluctuates. Untreated delirium may turn into a form of dementia. In pseudodementia, symptoms of depression are present and cognitive deficits are inconsistent and may vary from time to time. In addition, the patient is often aware of his or her deficit and shows appropriate concern about that. Dementia and depression can coexist in certain patients. As part of normal aging, it is likely that gradual decline in mental function, including memory, cognition, and abstract thinking, will be observed. In such instances, the degree and the extent of the impairment are proportionate to the age and are rarely of a profound nature. In amnestic disorder, the impairment is limited to short- and long-term memory, while other cognitive functions are within normal limits.

Diagnostic criteria of dementia, adapted from DSM-IV (1994) are outlined in Table 4.

Treatment and Prognosis

It is estimated that approximately 10% of all cases of dementia can be reversed while 25–30% can be stopped if specific treatment is initiated during the early stages. About 50–60% of all cases of dementia lack specific treatment (Wells, 1985). This fact underscores the importance of early detection, diagnosis, and treatment. Dementia that results from vitamin deficiency, for example, can be reversed completely when treated adequately with specific vitamins. On the other hand, several types of dementia do not respond, or respond minimally, to treatment, despite early detection. Examples include Alzheimer's disease and vascualr dementia. Several treatment modalities should be considered.

TABLE 4
DIAGNOSTIC CRITERIA FOR DEMENTIA
(Adapted from DSM-IV, 1994)

A. The development of multiple cognitive deficits including memory impairment, language disturbances, impairment in abstract thinking, impaired judgement and planning, and personality changes.

B. The symptoms are sufficient to interfere with work or social life, and represent a significant decline from a previous level of functioning.

C. The onset is insidious with ongoing gradual cognitive decline.

D. Not occurring during the course of delirium.

E. The condition is caused by an underlying brain disease, chronic general medical condition, or chronic substance abuse.

---

1. Treatment of Underlying Causes

It is always essential to identify the underlying medical illness or physical factor and provide specific treatment whenever possible. Such an approach offers the best chance for recovery. Early treatment is crucial in this regard, since any delay may allow the condition to worsen and create irreversible brain changes. For example, infectious processes may respond favorably to antibiotic treatment if treatment is provided during early stages. It is important to note here that the majority of medical disorders that cause dementia do not respond to treatment despite early diagnosis.

2. Pharmacologic Treatment

Recent research has shown that certain medication can be effective in the treatment of dementia. Cholinergic agents have been shown to slightly benefit certain populations of demented patients (Plotkin & Jarvik, 1986). Recently, the Food and Drug Adminstration (FDA) has approved the cholinergic agent tacrine hydrochloride (Cognex) for the treatment of Alzheimer's disease. Hydergine, a vasodilator, was shown in some instances to offer minimal improvement in demented patients; however, the significance of its benefit has been controversial (Jarvik, 1981). Methylphenidate (Ritalin) has been used, with some improvement, in certain demented patients who are also depressed. (Katon & Raskind, 1980). Other pharmacological agents such as antipsychotics, benzodiazepines, and antidepressants may be used for symptomatic treatment as clinically indicated.

3. Environmental Interventions

It is essential to assure the safety of demented patients since they are particularly vulnerable to dangerous situations due to their forgetfulness and disorientation. They are especially vulnerable to falls, bed sores, and medical complications. Adequate hygiene, and routine medical and dental care is important. Some patients may need to be institutionalized in nursing homes or other supervised settings. Maintaining familiar surroundings with daily routines and prominent display of clocks and calendars can be very helpful. Frequent contact with family members and easy access to radio, television, and newspapers help the patient remain aware of current events.

4. Family Support

Families of patients with dementia are subjected to significant stress and worries about their patients. Anger, resentment, hostility, guilt, and embarrassment are frequent emotional reactions. Educating family members about the nature, course, and prognosis of dementia is of particular importance. The availability of social and community resources is essential. Finally, counseling and family support groups can provide invaluable experience to most family members of demented patients.

Most cases of dementia follow a progressive and chronic course. Patients go through several stages before they become completely incapacitated. The prognosis varies depending on the nature of the underlying cause, the duration of the illness, and the effectiveness of the specific treatment.

II: AMNESTIC DISORDER

Amnestic disorder refers to a mental disorder that manifests primarily with memory disturbances. Both short-term memory and long-term memory are affected, while immediate recall is preserved. Recent memory is most impaired. Events from the distant past are better remembered than those of the more recent past (Wells, 1985). The level of consciousness is not impaired as in cases of delirium. In general, and unlike dementia, other cognitive functions are preserved in amnestic disorders. Confabulation can be striking, and the patient shows poor insight towards his or her deficit and exhibits a shallow affect.

The onset can be acute or insidious, depending on the cause. The course of the illness depends on the underlying etiology, but tends to be chronic.

This condition is caused mainly by thiamine deficiency that can be seen in the course of chronic alcoholism (Wernicke-Korsakoff syndrome) and malnutrition syndromes. It can also be caused by brain lesions involving temporal lobes, mammillary bodies, fornix and hippocampal areas. Such lesions can be produced by trauma, infection, anoxia, vascular accidents, tumors, and other pathological processes.

As in dementia, early identification and treatment of amnestic disorder is essential. Amnestic disorder should be differentiated from dementia, pseudodementia, normal aging, and psychogenic amnesia. In dementia, there is usually global impairment of most cognitive functions. In pseudodementia, symptoms of depression are present and mental status examination reveals inconsistent findings. In normal aging, the degree of memory loss is appropriate for age. In psychogenic amnesia, there is often severe psychological stress.

Certain cases of amnestic disorder are treatable and can be reversed. Treatment of the underlying physical factor is always critical. In cases of thiamine deficiency, treatment with that vitamin may offer dramatic results. However, advanced cases may show very little response. Prognosis is generally poor. Although memory defects tend to improve with time, very few patients show full recovery.

4

PSYCHOTIC DISORDERS DUE TO MEDICAL CONDITIONS

I. DELUSIONAL DISORDER DUE TO MEDICAL CONDITIONS

Clinical Features

Delusional disorder can be induced by an underlying medical illness or by substance abuse. Delusions can mimic those encountered in "primary" psychiatric disorders and may include paranoid, jealous, or somatic types. Often, the delusions are firmly held by the patient and can not be shaken by reasoning. However, in certain cases, the delusions can be fleeting and changeable. Typically, the patient does not show any changes in the level of consciousness as in the case of delirium. Mild cognitive impairment may be present in association with the disorder. Hallucinatory symptoms may be present, but they rarely dominate the clinical picture.

It is important to note here that it is not uncommon to see several psychiatric symptoms occurring simultaneously as a result of a single physical condition. For example, intoxication with marijuana can cause paranoid delusions, hallucinations, anxiety, and depression at the same time. In addition, and depending on the underlying medical condition, other physical and neurological signs and symptoms are likely to be present as well.

Clinical Examples

CASE ONE: A 22-year-old college student was seen in the emergency room due to a sudden onset of paranoid delusions consisting of fear of being followed by two men who he believed were waiting outside the hospital in order to kill him. Urine and blood examination showed traces of cocaine and marijuana. Treatment consisted of small doses of haloperidol for several days with dramatic results.

CASE TWO: A 75-year-old man was seen in the psychiatrist's office because of gradual onset of delusions of jealousy. The patient believed that his 77-year-old wife was having an affair with a young man. Although the story could not be substantiated by the patient or any family member, he insisted on his accusations and demanded a divorce. Clinical evaluation and head CT scan revealed a tumor of the pituitary gland. The patient refused to be treated until physical symptoms developed.

The course of psychotic disorders resulting from medical conditions or substance abuse varies depending on the underlying cause. It can be short and may resolve without any residual symptoms, as in the case of drug intoxication. Or it may become chronic with progressive symptoms that may not improve despite treatment, as in the case of cerebrovascular accidents.

Etiology and Pathophysiology

Theoretically, any physical illness that may affect the brain directly or indirectly can produce a delusional disorder. It is believed that physical conditions influence certain neurotransmitters, and consequently produce corresponding psychiatric symptoms. Intoxication with drugs and pharmacological agents is the most common factor leading to delusional disorder compared to other physical causes. Amphetamine is believed to be one of the major offenders in this regard. Other drugs include similar CNS stimulants, cocaine, LSD, marijuana, L-dopa preparations, bromocriptine, corticosteroids, and others. Lesions of the right cerebral hemisphere, especially those involving the right parietal lobe, can cause a peculiar form of delusional disorder in which the patient denies his or her paralysis (Well, 1985). Other causes include metabolic and endocrine disorders, encephalitis, head trauma, brain tumors, strokes, Huntington's chorea, and temporal lobe epilepsy.

Differential Diagnosis and Diagnostic Criteria

Delusional disorder due to medical conditions and substance abuse should be differentiated from delusions encountered in "primary" psychiatric disorders such as schizophrenia, delusional disorder, or mood disorders. These illnesses have specific diagnostic criteria which can aid in making the differential diagnosis. It should also be differentiated from delusions that occur in the course of delirium where the level of consciousness is variable, and from delusions that develop in the course of dementia where intellectual abilities are significantly compromised.

Diagnostic criteria are outlined in Table 5.

Treatment and Prognosis

Treatment of delusional disorder should be directed at the underlying cause. In cases of intoxication with drugs such as amphetamine or cocaine, cessation of the drug can eliminate the condition. Occasionally, antipsychotic medication or benzodiazepines may be needed. In cases of side effects to medications such as Inderal or Digoxin, reduction in the dosage or substitution with another agent may be sufficient. If dose reduction or drug substitution is not feasible, antipsychotic medication can be used with good results.

TABLE 5
DIAGNOSTIC CRITERIA FOR PSYCHOTIC
DISORDER DUE TO MEDICAL CONDITIONS OR
SUBSTANCE ABUSE
(Adapted from DSM-IV, 1994)

A. Prominent hallucinations or delusions.

B. The presence of an underlying medical condition, a history of drug ingestion or withdrawal, or medication use that is believed to be etiologically related to the disturbance.

C. The disturbance is not occurring exclusively during delirium.

D. The disturbance is not caused by another mental disorder.

Most cases of delusional disorder due to medical conditions or substance abuse respond well to treatment and are short-lived. However, conditions that result from ongoing brain disorder such as multiple sclerosis or Huntington's chorea may be progressive and respond to no treatment. In all instances, antipsychotic medications can still be used with favorable outcome. Epileptic disorders may respond well to Tegretol or other antiepileptic agents.

Supportive psychotherapy may be indicated in certain chronic cases in which preexisting personality and psychodynamic factors influence the clinical presentation and the course of the illness.

II. HALLUCINOSIS

Definition and Clinical Features

Hallucinosis refers to hallucinatory symptoms that occur in a clear state of consciousness and in the absence of any "primary" psychiatric condition. Hallucinations can involve all sensory modalities and present with various auditory, visual, tactile, olfactory, and gustatory percep- tions. Typically, hallucinatory symptoms are of the simple unformed variety, but complex hallucinations are not uncommon. Visual hallucinations are encountered most frequently in "organic" conditions. Examples include side effects to pharmacological agents and cerebrovascu- lar accidents. Auditory hallucinations occur frequently in cases of alcohol hallucinosis and can mimic to a large extent those of schizophrenic disorders. Tactile halluci- nations are seen commonly in cases of alcohol withdrawal and drug intoxication. Olfactory and gustatory hallucina- tions are seen most frequently in cases of temporal lobe epilepsy (Asaad, 1990).

The patient is usually alert and is aware of the unreality of his or her perceptions. Other psychiatric symptoms can accompany hallucinosis, including delusions, anxiety, depression, and cognitive impairment. Physical and neu- rological symptoms may be present depending on the underlying medical illness.

Clinical Examples

CASE ONE: A 74-year-old man was seen in consultation while he was in the hospital for treatment of cardiac failure. The patient reported having visual hallucinations that consisted of flames that were coming from under chairs in his room. Clinical evaluation confirmed that the onset of his hallucinations coincided with an increase in the dosage of Digoxin. Hallucinations disappeared when Digoxin was discontinued and replaced by another drug.

CASE TWO: A 51-year-old woman was seen in the emer- gency room complaining of persistent auditory hallucina- tions consisting of voices of several people insulting her and telling her to kill herself. A complete history revealed that the patient had a significant history of alcohol abuse and that she had stopped drinking several days earlier.

Treatment consisted of small doses of haloperidol, with moderate improvement.

Etiology and Pathophysiology

Hallucinosis occurs mainly as side effects to various pharmacological agents or as a result of drug intoxication. Alcohol withdrawal causes alcohol hallucinosis, as indicated above. Other conditions that can cause hallucinosis include metabolic and endocrine disorders, cerebrovascular disorders, degenerative brain disorders, infections, and epileptic disorders. Alcohol hallucinosis is discussed in Chapter Sixteen.

It is believed that changes in the levels of neurotransmitters in the brain may be responsible for hallucinatory symptoms. It has been shown that an increase in dopamine level or a decrease in serotonin level may be associated with the emergence of hallucinatory symptoms (Asaad, 1990).

Differential Diagnosis and Diagnostic Criteria

Hallucinosis should be differentiated from hallucinations that occur in delirium, schizophrenia, mania, depression, and hysteria. In delirium, the level of consciousness is clouded and variable. In "primary" psychiatric disorders, other symptoms are often present and the clinical course is different.

Diagnostic criteria are provided in Table 5.

Treatment and Prognosis

Treatment of hallucinosis should be aimed at the underlying causative factor. For example, the discontinuation of a certain medication or a drug may be sufficient in certain cases. Treatment of specific medical illnesses that may be causing hallucinatory symptoms is usually helpful. In all circumstances, the use of small doses of an antipsychotic agent can be highly beneficial. Supportive psychotherapy is often helpful as well.

Most cases of hallucinosis are acute and short-lived. However, certain conditions may become chronic and show little response to treatment. This is particularly true for hallucinations that are caused by underlying medical conditions that are not amenable to treatment, such as Alzheimer's disease and vascular dementia.

5

MOOD DISORDER AND ANXIETY DISORDER DUE TO MEDICAL CONDITIONS

I. MOOD DISORDER

Clinical Features

Mood disorder consisting of any depressive or manic condition can be caused by an underlying medical illness or substance abuse. Depressive symptoms may be mild or severe, and may not be easily distinguished from those seen in "primary" depressive illness. Symptoms include sleep and appetite disturbances, low energy level, poor concentration, lack of interest in pleasurable activities, hopelessness, helplessness, and suicidal ideation. Manic symptoms include increased energy level, diminished need for sleep, racing thoughts, pressured speech, and inflated self-worth. Physical and specific neurological symptoms may be present depending on the underlying causative factors.

The onset may be sudden or gradual and the course can be limited or chronic depending on the medical condition.

Patients tend to show good insight and significant concern regarding their emotional state.

Clinical Examples

CASE ONE: A 47-year-old male was referred by his internist to the psychiatrist because of history of depressive symptoms that included insomnia, poor appetite, fatigue, poor concentration, low energy level, and a sense of hopelessness. The symptoms lasted for several months and became progressively worse. Treatment with antidepressants offered slight improvement. Several weeks later, the patient developed jaundice and back pain when sleeping on his back. Clinical investigations revealed the presence of pancreatic cancer that was thought to have been responsible for the depressive symptoms.

CASE TWO: A 43-year-old woman was seen in the hospital while she was being treated with Prednisone for multiple sclerosis. She was experiencing racing thoughts, pressured speech, increased energy level, and grandiose delusions. The symptoms subsided after Prednisone therapy was concluded. The diagnosis of manic disorder secondary to Prednisone treatment was made.

Etiology and Pathophysiology

Mood disorders are caused more often by drugs or pharmacological agents than by physical factors. Cocaine, amphetamines and other stimulants, corticosteroids, and antidepressant medications are capable of producing hypomanic or even manic states. Alcohol, barbiturates, benzodiazepines, corticosteroids, levodopa, antihypertensive medications such as reserpine, methyldopa, and propranolol are known to induce depressive conditions.

In addition, other conditions that affect the brain directly or indirectly can cause mood disorder. Depression has been reported to occur as a result of hypothyroidism, Cushing's syndrome, influenza, infectious mononucleosis, pernicious anemia, carcinoma of the pancreas, brain tumors, systemic lupus erythematosus, strokes (particularly those of the left hemisphere), Huntington's disease, Parkinson's disease, and epilepsy. Manic symptoms have been reported in cases of multiple sclerosis, neurosyphilis, and strokes of the right hemisphere (Lipowski, 1980a; Wells, 1985).

The exact mechanism by which physical conditions can cause mood changes is not completely known. However, it is believed that such physical factors may alter the levels of norepinephrine and serotonin within the brain and, consequently, create mood changes. Other neurotransmitters may be involved as well (Yudofsky & Hales, 1992).

Differential Diagnosis and Diagnostic Criteria

Mood disorder due to medical conditions and substance abuse should be differentiated from "primary" depressive disorders and bipolar disorders. Family history, past history, course, and associated clinical features can help in making the diagnosis. It is important to note here that other "organic" mental disorders such as hallucinosis and delusional disorder can accompany mood disorder. The diagnosis cannot be made when depressive or manic symptoms occur along with changes in the level of consciousness during the course of delirium.

Diagnostic criteria for mood disorder due to medical conditions or substance abuse are outlined in Table 6.

Treatment and Prognosis

Treatment of mood disorders should be directed at the underlying medical condition or the responsible drug or medication. In addition, traditional treatment with antidepressants, lithium, and other psychotropic medication can be highly effective. Psychotherapy may be needed on a short-term basis for education and support.

TABLE 6
DIAGNOSTIC CRITERIA FOR MOOD
DISORDER DUE TO MEDICAL CONDITIONS
OR SUBSTANCE ABUSE
(Adapted from DSM-IV, 1994)

A. Prominent and persistent depressed or elevated mood.

B. The presence of an underlying medical condition, a history of drug ingestion or withdrawal, or medication use that is believed to be etiologically related to the disturbance.

C. The disturbance is not occurring exclusively during delirium.

D. The disturbance is not caused by another mental disorder.

E. The condition causes sufficient distress and interferes with the patient's social or occupational life.

The prognosis is generally good, provided the underlying medical illness is corrected. In cases where such treatment is not effective, mood disorder may take a chronic course.

II. ANXIETY DISORDER

Clinical Features

Symptoms of generalized anxiety, panic attacks, obsessions, or compulsions can be caused by medical conditions or substance abuse. The symptoms are similar to those seen in "primary" generalized anxiety disorder, panic disorder, and obsessive-compulsive disorder, respectively. Physical and neurological symptoms may be present depending on the underlying cause.

As in other "organic" conditions, the onset may be sudden or gradual depending on the cause, and the course depends on the outcome of the treatment for the specific underlying condition.

Clinical Examples

CASE ONE: A 52-year-old woman complained of symptoms of anxiety with palpitations, shortness of breath, perspiration, and fear of dying. Clinical evaluation revealed a toxic nodule in the thyroid gland. Surgical removal of the tumor resulted in complete remission of anxiety symptoms.

CASE TWO: A 49-year-old man was referred by the psychiatrist back to the internist for further medical evaluation concerning episodes of severe anxiety that would be accompanied at times with severe headache and lightheadedness. A thorough evaluation showed a pheochromocytoma (a tumor of the adrenal gland that secretes norepinephrine). Surgical removal of the tumor resulted in complete remission of the symptoms.

Etiology and Pathophysiology

The most common medical causes of anxiety disorders include endocrine disorders, especially the thyroid and the adrenal glands, and fasting hypoglycemia. Drugs such as cocaine and amphetamine can lead to anxiety symptoms. Certain pharmacological agents such as antidepressants can lead to such symptoms as well. Withdrawal from alcohol and sedatives can precipitate anxiety states. Other causes include brain tumors in the vicinity of the third ventricle, epilepsy, pulmonary embolus, aspirin intolerance, and brucellosis. It is believed that changes in levels of neurotransmitters are responsible for the clinical manifestations of anxiety symptoms.

Differential Diagnosis and Diagnostic Criteria

Anxiety disorders due to medical conditions or substance abuse should be differentiated from "primary" generalized anxiety disorder, panic disorder, and obsessive-compulsive disorder. Past history, family history, clinical presentation, and the presence of associated features can be of great help. Other mental disorders such as mood disorder may accompany anxiety disorder. The diagnosis can not be made when anxiety occurs during the course of delirium in which the level of consciousness may vary.

The diagnostic criteria of anxiety disorder due to medical conditions or substance abuse are outlined in Table 7.

TABLE 7
DIAGNOSTIC CRITERIA FOR ANXIETY
DISORDER DUE TO MEDICAL CONDITIONS
OR SUBSTANCE ABUSE
(Adapted from DSM-IV, 1994)

A.   Prominent and recurrent generalized anxiety, panic attacks, obsessions, or compulsions.

B.   The presence of an underlying medical condition, a history of drug ingestion or withdrawal, or medication use that is believed to be etiologically related to the disturbance.

C.   The disturbance is not occurring exclusively during delirium

D.   The disturbance is not caused by another mental disorder.

E.   The condition causes sufficient distress and interferes with the patient's social or occupational life.

Treatment and Prognosis

As in other "organic" mental disorders, it is always essential to identify and treat the underlying medical condition or eliminate the substance or medication that may be responsible for the anxiety state. However, the use of benzodiazepines and other medications may be necessary until specific treatment is implemented.

The prognosis is generally favorable whenever the underlying condition is treatable. Otherwise, anxiety may persist and symptomatic treatment may need to be carried out on a long-term basis.

6

PERSONALITY CHANGE DUE TO MEDICAL CONDITIONS

CLINICAL FEATURES

Personality change including behavioral and characterological disturbances can develop as a result of a wide variety of medical conditions. The changes may represent an accentuation of previously characteristic traits or the onset of new traits. Most common symptoms include mood instability, recurrent outbursts of aggression or rage, impairment in social judgement, apathy and indifference, and suspiciousness or paranoid ideation. Frequently, the patient begins to show signs of social disinhibition and inappropriate sexual behavior.

Family members and friends may notice the changes early on and before they become evident to the examiner. The patient generally ignores criticism concerning his or her inappropriate behavior, or at best, minimizes its significance. As the condition progresses, the behavior becomes grossly inappropriate, and the patient is likely to get into trouble as a result. In severe cases, and when treatment is not effective, the patient can pose danger to self or others and may require to be institutionalized.

Although the majority of cases are encountered during adult life, the disorder can develop at any age, including childhood. In such instances, the parents may notice progressive changes in the child's usual behavior patterns. The child may become withdrawn and irritable. He or she may lose interest in social activities, and fall behind in school work.

Other psychiatric symptoms, including depression, anxiety, and cognitive limitations, can accompany the disorder. When such symptoms are severe enough, appropriate diagnoses can be made in addition to personality change. Furthermore, neurological and physical symptoms may be present depending on the organic etiology.

CASE EXAMPLES

CASE ONE: A 37-year-old man, who was previously described as shy and highly polite, was evaluated by the psychiatrist at the request of his employer because of sudden onset of behavior that involved making inappropriate sexual remarks towards several female employees on several occasions. Complete medical evaluation which included a CAT scan of the brain revealed a meningioma pressing on the frontal lobe. Surgical removal of the tumor resulted in gradual resolution of the symptoms. Within a few weeks, the patient returned to his normal pattern of behavior.

CASE TWO: A 22-year-old woman who was known for her calm and friendly manner began exhibiting frequent outbursts of rage and violent episodes during which she would attack others and destroy property. A complete neurological work-up, including an EEG, showed the presence of Temporal Lobe Epilepsy. The patient was treated with Tegretol, an antiepileptic agent, which resulted in significant improvement in her condition.

CASE THREE: A 17-year-old high school student became increasingly withdrawn and indifferent. He quit his sports activities and fell behind in his school work. He became highly suspicious and lost most of his friends. When the behavior was clearly evident to his family and teachers, a psychiatric evaluations was conducted. Although the diagnosis of schizophrenia was suspected, a complete medical work-up was pursued. Urine analysis showed high levels of marijuana. Further history revealed that he had been abusing the drug for at least a year. The diagnosis of personality change secondary to marijuana abuse was made. Reversal of most symptoms occurred following the cessation of the use of the drug. Drug rehabilitation and Narcotics Anonymous (NA) meetings were effective in maintaining the improvement over the following several months.

ETIOLOGY AND PATHOPHYSIOLOGY

Personality change can be caused by almost any of the factors that have been listed previously in connection with other "organic" mental disorders. Most commonly, the disorder occurs as a result of closed head injuries. Typically, personality change begins to emerge after all physical symptoms have subsided. The disorder occurs more often following traumatic lesions of the frontal or temporal lobes. Personality changes are more pronounced after bilateral traumatic lesions involving the frontal lobes (Wells, 1985). Other causes include tumors and strokes involving the frontal lobe area. Temporal Lobe Epilepsy can be responsible for an explosive variety of organic personality disorders. Multiple sclerosis, Huntington's chorea, Wilson's disease, Cushing's syndrome, and chronic heavy ingestion of marijuana represent less frequent causes (Spar, 1989).

DIFFERENTIAL DIAGNOSIS AND DIAGNOSTIC CRITERIA

Personality change needs to be differentiated from other mental disorders such as delirium by the absence of changes in the level of consciousness, and from dementia by the absence of significant cognitive impairment. It is important to note here that, in some instances, personality change may signal the onset of dementia, which may later evolve and eventually dominate the clinical picture. Occasionally, personality change may be accompanied by other mental disorders such as hallucinosis, mood disorder, and delusional disorder.

Personality change due to medical conditions may need to be differentiated from "primary" psychiatric disorders which involve certain characterological changes. These include schizophrenia, mood disorders, delusional disorders, impulse control disorders that are not attributed to physical factors, personality disorders, and substance abuse disorders.

The diagnostic criteria of personality change due to medical conditions are outlined in Table 8.

TREATMENT AND PROGNOSIS

Treatment of personality change due to medical conditions should be aimed at the underlying problem. However, the use of psychotropic medications may be essential. Antipsychotic, antidepressant and antianxiety agents can be used as needed depending on the clinical presentation. Explosive personality disorder, which may be caused by temporal lobe epilepsy and other factors, may respond favorably to anticonvulsant medications such as Tegretol and Depakote. Lithium and propranolol have also been used effectively in such cases. Behavioral therapies and supportive psychotherapy can be effective in combination with psychotropic medications. Family support and education are also important.

TABLE 8
DIAGNOSTIC CRITERIA FOR PERSONALITY CHANGE
DUE TO MEDICAL CONDITIONS
(Adapted from DSM-IV, 1994)

A. A persistent personality disturbance that reflects a change from a previous pattern of behavior.

B. The presence of an underlying medical condition that is believed to be etiologically related to the disturbance.

C. The disturbance is not occurring exclusively during delirium and does not meet criteria for dementia.

D. The disturbance is not caused by another mental disorder.

E. The condition causes sufficient distress and interferes with the patient's social or occupational life.

The course depends on the etiology and outcome of the treatment of the underlying illness. Cases that result from permanent brain damage are likely to become long-standing disorders. Examples include multiple sclerosis and serious traumatic brain injuries. The degree of impairment is variable and depends on the site and the extent of brain lesion.

Patients with personality change due to medical conditions may present danger to themselves or others due to their poor judgment, impulsivity, or explosive behavior. In such instances, institutionalization or closely supervised settings may be needed.

7

ALZHEIMER'S DISEASE AND OTHER DEGENERATIVE DEMENTIAS

As indicated earlier, dementia can be caused by a wide variety of neurological and other medical conditions. In this chapter, we will discuss several specific syndromes that involve progressive degenerative illnesses that, among other signs and symptoms, present with dementia.

ALZHEIMER'S DISEASE

Definition and Clinical Manifestations

Alzheimer's disease refers to a specific progressive degenerative disorder of the neurons of the cerebral cortex. Consequently, cognitive deficits as well as personality changes develop depending on the extent of the neuronal degeneration. Alzheimer's disease is believed to be the single most common dementing disease of the elderly. The disease usually strikes people between ages 40 and 90, and equally afflicts men and women. It is estimated that

51

between two and four million people suffer from this illness in the United States alone. The disease is progressive, and patients are expected to survive approximately 10 years from the time of the initial diagnosis until death, which may be caused by several complications (Cummings, 1992).

The onset is usually insidious, and early deficits can be noticed only by close relatives. As the illness progresses, symptoms become obvious to most observers. The patient may lose insight into the changes at an early stage and show very little concern regarding his or her cognitive deficits. This often makes it easier for the patient to cope with the illness, yet may create more problems for the family and other caretakers.

Three phases are generally observed. During the first phase, which may last from two to three years, the patient shows signs of impaired memory, disorientation, and difficulties in performing everyday tasks. The second phase is characterized by rapid deterioration of cognitive functions and the onset of remarkable personality changes. Focal neurological signs and symptoms may develop. Hallucinations, delusions, mood changes, and behavioral disturbances are common. The third or terminal phase consists of profound apathy and decrease in psychomotor activity. The patient becomes bedridden and incontinent of urine and feces. Gross neurological disabilities and epilepsy may develop. The patient is usually unable to feed himself or herself and will eventually require total nursing care (Lishman, 1987).

Etiology and Pathophysiology

Alzheimer's disease is caused by progressive neuronal degeneration of the cerebral cortex, leading to cortical atrophy. The pathological burden of the disease is greatest in the medial aspects of the temporal lobe, the posterior cingulate region, and the temporal-parietal junction. The frontal cortex is less affected by the disease. In addition to neuronal loss, microscopic examination of the cortical tissue reveals gliosis, senile plaques, neurofibrillary tangles, and granulovascular degeneration. Neurotransmitter changes include marked reduction in choline acetyltransferase and somatostatin, and to a lesser extent a decrease in the levels of serotonin, GABA, and norepinephrine (Cummings, 1992).

The exact cause of Alzheimer's disease remains unknown. Several hypotheses have been proposed. The cholinergic theory remains the most likely one as evidenced by research findings. According to this theory, the disease can be caused by deficit in the cholinergic system in the cerebral cortex. Other hypotheses have proposed an infective process, immunological factors, and toxicity from aluminum as possible etiological factors in the production of Alzheimer's disease (Lishman, 1987). To date, no definitive conclusion has been reached.

It has been shown that Down's syndrome predisposes to Alzheimer's disease, and that first degree biologic relatives of people with presenile (before age 65) onset of Alzheimer's disease are more likely to develop dementia compared to the general population. In addition, it has been shown that Alzheimer's disease can be inherited as a dominant trait.

Diagnosis and Differential Diagnosis

The diagnosis of Alzheimer's disease is often made based on clinical grounds. The patient has to meet the diagnostic criteria for dementia (see Table 4). In addition, the onset of Alzheimer's disease is always insidious, and the course is progressive. Other specific causes of dementia must be excluded before this diagnosis is made.

Laboratory investigations may be pursued to clarify the diagnosis and exclude other conditions. Most laboratory studies remain normal in patients with Alzheimer's diseases. Computerized tomography and MRI of the brain may reveal cerebral atrophy with widened cortical sulci and enlarged cerebral ventricles. Electroencephalographic studies may show generalized slowing, with abnormalities in the parietal lobes. Positron emission tomography (PET) reveals a characteristic pattern of hypometabolism, with diminished glucose utilization in the parietal lobes and, eventually, in the frontal lobes. Single- photon emission-computed tomography (SPECT) shows decrease in blood flow in the parietal and posterior temporal lobes of both hemispheres of most patients with Alzheimer's disease (Cummings, 1992).

Alzheimer's disease should be differentiated from the normal process of aging, vascular dementia, major depression in the elderly, and other specific "organic" mental disorders that can cause corresponding dementia syndromes. In the normal process of aging, cognitive deficits are mild and are appropriate for age. In vascular dementia, cognitive deficit is often variable, and focal neurologic signs exist along with evidence of vascular disease.

Major depression in the elderly can present with pseudodementia and may mimic Alzheimer's disease. In such instances, the cognitive deficit is inconsistent and the patient is aware of his or her deficits and is distressed by them. Symptoms of major depression are present in pseudodementia, but Alzheimer's disease and major depression can occur simultaneously. Other specific causes of dementia such as subdural hematoma, normal pressure hydrocephalus, cerebral neoplasms, Parkinson's disease, vitamin B12 deficiency, hypothyroidism, drug intoxication, and others can be ruled out on the basis history, physical examination, and appropriate laboratory investigations (DSM-IV, 1994).

Treatment and Prognosis

1. Pharmacological Treatments

To date, there is no specific drug that is capable of providing significant relief of Alzheimer's symptoms. Several experimental medications have been tried. Based on the cholinergic theory, which speculates that Alzheimer's disease may be caused by deficiency in the cholinergic system, several cholinergic agents have been used with variable results and moderate improvement in some cases. These include choline, lecithin, arecholine and physostigmine. As indicated earlier, the cholinergic agent tacrine hydrochloride (Cognex) has been approved by the FDA for clinical use for Alzhemer's disease. Vasodilators such as Hydergine have also been tried, with controversial conclusions. The argument that supports their possible effectiveness is based on the fact that vasodilators improve blood perfusion in the cortical areas and, consequently, improve the metabolism, the synthesis, and the release of acetylcholine in the brain. Agents that enhance the concentration of neurotransmitters, such as serotonin, norepinephrine, and dopamine, have demonstrated some effectiveness, as well. These include tricyclic antidepressants, monoamine oxidase inhibitors, tryptophan, D-Amphetamine, Ritalin, clonidine, and L-Dopa (Meyers & Young, 1989).

It is important to emphasize here that various psychotropic medications can be used effectively to control symptoms of agitation, psychosis, depression, or anxiety that may occur in association with Alzheimer's disease.

2. Family Education and Support

It is particularly difficult for family members to learn that their loved spouse, parent, or grandparent suffers from Alzheimer's disease and soon may not be able to remember important events or even recognize family members. Educating the family about the nature of the illness, its course, and prognosis is essential. In some instances, family support groups and psychotherapy may be needed. Most patients who suffer from Alzheimer's disease are cared for at home, especially during the early phase of the illness. It is important to emphasize the fact that such patients require close supervision due to the possibility of subjecting themselves or others to dangerous situations. Patients with Alzheimer's disease have the tendency to wander and get lost away from home. They also may cause fires or other serious accidents due to their forgetfulness and poor judgment. Patients with serious medical problems may require skilled nursing care while still living at home.

3. Institutionalization

The decision to place a parent or a spouse into a nursing home is always difficult. The sense of guilt often interferes with making such decisions. However, sooner or later the family may no longer be able to provide the appropriate level of care that the patient requires, and will realize that placing the patient in a nursing home would be in his or her best interest. Most patients who are placed in nursing homes or other supervised settings react with anxiety and depression initially. Later, as they settle and get used to the new environment, they become more comfortable and may get involved in various programs and activities that are available.

As indicated earlier, Alzheimer's disease is progressive and irreversible. Complications include bed sores, infections, and strokes. Death often occurs as a result of such complications.

PICK'S DISEASE

Definition and Clinical Features

Pick's disease is a progressive degenerative dementia that involves mainly the frontal lobe and the anterior portion of the temporal lobe. Consequently, symptoms of dementia are those of frontal lobe syndrome nature in which the patient is often disinhibited and shows poor judgment, followed by impairment in memory and intellect. The disease is less common than Alzheimer's disease, and women are affected almost twice frequently as men. The age of onset is mostly between 50 and 60, although some cases have been reported in people in their 20s. Personality changes and social impairment often precede impairment in memory and intellect. Common symptoms include inappropriate sexual behavior, stealing, alcoholism, and ill-judged social conduct. The individual's insight is often severely impaired from the early stages. Patients may appear euphoric or apathic (Lishman, 1987). In addition, all other symptoms associated with dementia can occur (see Table 4 and Chapter Three). Focal neurological signs and symptoms may be observed as well.

Etiology and Pathophysiology

The disease is thought to be genetic, and may be inherited through a single autosomal dominant gene; however, most cases appear to arise sporadically. Some researchers have found increased concentration of zinc in the brain and red blood cells of patients with Pick's disease. Other studies failed to show cholinergic brain deficit typical of Alzheimer's disease. EEG studies show lower incidence of abnormalities compared to Alzheimer's disease. CT scan of the brain in typical cases shows marked atrophy in the anterior portions of the frontal and temporal lobes, with enlargement of the frontal horns. Microscopic examination of affected cortical areas shows neuronal loss along with dense proliferation of astrocytes and fibrous gliosis. Characteristic Pick bodies may be seen inside swollen neurons (Lishman, 1987).

Differential Diagnosis

Pick's disease should be distinguished from Alzheimer's disease by its relative earlier onset, by the appearance of personality changes and social disinhibition before impairment in memory and intellect, and by frontal lobe atrophy that can be documented by CT scan and MRI of the brain. It should also be distinguished from all other causes of dementia and pseudodementia as discussed above in the section of Alzheimer's disease.

Treatment and Prognosis

There is no specific treatment for Pick's disease. However, clinical management is similar to that of Alzheimer's disease. Cholinergic agents are not indicated for Pick's disease, and vasodilators have limited value. Psychotropic medications can be used along the same guidelines used with Alzheimer's disease. Family education and support are essential, and institutionalization is almost inevitable.

The prognosis is guarded, and death usually occurs due to complications similar to those of Alzheimer's disease.

PARKINSON'S DISEASE

Definition and Clinical Features

Parkinson's disease is a degenerative brain disease that affects the basal ganglia and causes movement disorder, dementia, and psychiatric symptoms. It is estimated that about one million individuals in North America are affected by this illness. The prevalence of this disease increases dramatically with age, especially after age 65. Dementia occurs in 10%–30%, and depression occurs in 15%–30% of all patients with Parkinson's disease (Whitehouse, Friedland & Straus, 1992).

Motor dysfunction consists of tremor which mostly involves the hands, muscle rigidity, poverty and slowness of movement, lack of facial expression, and small-stepped shuffling gait.

The majority of patients with Parkinson's disease suffer from a certain degree of cognitive impairment. As the disease progresses, severe dementia develops. Two different types of dementia have been described (Addonizio,

1989): cortical dementia and subcortical dementia. The cortical type presents with symptoms similar to Alzheimer's disease. The subcortical type presents with forgetfulness, while preserving the ability to learn new material, and apathy. Eventually, subcortical dementia leads to severe cognitive deficit similar to the cortical type.

Psychiatric symptoms associated with Parkinson's disease include mood disorders, psychosis, and personality changes. Major depression and dysthymia are most common, especially in patients with early onset Parkinson's disease. Less commonly, patients report symptoms of anxiety and phobias (Whitehouse et al., 1992). Psychotic symptoms of a schizophrenic nature have been reported in patients with Parkinson's disease in the absence of pharmacological treatment (Mjones, 1949). However, most psychotic symptoms, including hallucinations and delusions, occur as a result of treatment of Parkinson's disease with L-Dopa preparations and other dopaminergic agents. Personality changes may include irritability, suspiciousness, and exaggeration of premorbid personality traits.

Etiology and Pathophysiology

Parkinson's disease results from progressive degeneration of the basal ganglia in the brain, leading to reduction in the dopaminergic function. The majority of cases are of an idiopathic etiology where no specific causes could be found. However, the disease can be produced by other pathological conditions that cause damage to the basal ganglia. These include cerebral trauma, encephalitis, and cerebrovascular disorders. In addition, Parkinsonian symptoms may result from the administration of dopamine blocking agents such as antipsychotic medications, and from intoxication with carbon monoxide and heavy metals (Addonizio, 1989).

The correlation between neuronal degeneration observed in the basal ganglia of patients with Parkinson's disease and the onset of dementia and psychiatric symptoms remains unclear. However, it has been reported that some patients with symptoms of dementia develop senile plaques and neurofibrillary tangles identical to those found in Alzheimer's disease, while others show loss of cortical cholinergic markers. The onset of psychiatric symptoms may correlate with changes in the levels of neurotransmitters such as serotonin, norepinephrine, and corticotropin releasing factor (Whitehouse et al., 1992).

Differential Diagnosis

Motor dysfunction in Parkinson's disease needs to be differentiated from other neurological conditions that can cause similar symptoms. Complete neurological examination and appropriate diagnostic investigations are often helpful.

Dementia in the course of Parkinson's disease should be differentiated from Alzheimer's disease and other types of dementia, including Pick's diseases, vascular dementia, and alcohol-related dementia.

Depression in the course of Parkinson's disease needs to be differentiated from major depression and other depressive disorders. Hallucinations and delusions are rare in untreated Parkinson's disease. However, symptoms arising from treatment with L-dopa preparations should be differentiated from other psychotic conditions.

Treatment and Prognosis

Treatment of Parkinson's disease consists mainly of administering dopamine agonists that increase the level of dopamine in the basal ganglia. Such agents include L-dopa, amantadine, and bromocriptine. Anticholinergic agents may be used in conjunction with dopamine agonists.

Treatment with such preparations often causes the emergence of psychotic reactions, especially visual and auditory hallucinations. When these psychotic symptoms are treated with antipsychotic agents, the effect of antiparkinsonian agents is reduced, since antipsychotic agents block dopamine receptors. The use of clozapine to treat psychosis in Parkinson's disease has been shown to be successful without diminishing the effect of the antiparkinsonian agents (Friedman & Lannon, 1989). Benzodiazepines may be used to treat agitation and psychotic reactions with some success.

Dementia in the course of Parkinson's disease is treated along the same guidelines for the treatment of Alzheimer's disease.

Depression in the course of Parkinson's disease must be treated aggressively. Antidepressants along with psychotherapy can be highly effective. Occasionally, electroconvulsive therapy may be needed.

The prognosis is somewhat guarded due to the progressive nature of the disease. The rate of progression and the degree of the disability vary a great deal from one patient to another. When treated properly, depression has a good prognosis. Dementia is always progressive and has a guarded prognosis. The mortality rate in patients with Parkinson's disease is three times that of the general population. Common causes of death include cardiac and cerebral vascular disease, infections, and tumors (Lishman, 1987).

HUNTINGTON'S DISEASE

Definition and Clinical Features

Huntington's disease refers to a progressive genetic illness that manifests with abnormal movements, psychiatric symptoms, and dementia. The illness can strike at any time. However, it is most likely to occur during the fourth and fifth decades of life. It has been estimated that the prevalence rate among Caucasians is between 5 and 7 cases per 100,000, with considerable differences among ethnic groups (Folstein, 1989).

Both involuntary movements and abnormal voluntary movements occur in Huntington's disease. The classic abnormality consists of chorea, a sudden jerky movement of the limbs, trunk, or face. Other abnormalities in muscle movements may be observed.

Cognitive deficits appear early in the course of Huntington's disease and may precede movement abnormalities. Deficits in memory and verbal fluency occur during rather early stages. Other forms of cognitive impairment develop with the progression of the disease.

Psychiatric symptoms may also precede movement abnormalities and usually include depression, irritability, anxiety, apathy, and hallucinations. Certain psychiatric disorders were found to occur more frequently in patients with Huntington's disease. These disorders include major depression, bipolar disorder, schizophreniform disorder, atypical psychosis, and intermittent explosive disorder (Folstein, 1989).

Etiology and Pathophysiology

The disease is transmitted genetically as an autosomal dominant trait. It is believed that the gene for Huntington's disease is located on chromosome 4. Genetic testing of family members of patients with the disease is now possible for the purpose of identifying those who are at risk (Gusella et al., 1983).

It has been suggested that the symptoms of Huntington's disease occur because of alterations in the concentration and relative balance among several neurotransmitters in the basal ganglia. The neurotransmitters involved include GABA and acetylcholine (Folstein, 1989).

In addition to the degeneration and atrophy that take place in the basal ganglia, similar atrophy occurs in the prefrontal and frontal cortical areas, which may account for the cognitive dysfunction encountered in the disease (Whitehouse et al., 1992).

Differential Diagnosis

Due to the relatively common occurrence of psychiatric symptoms as part of Huntington's disease, the illness needs to be differentiated from psychiatric disorders such as major depression, schizophrenia and other psychotic conditions, and personality disorders. The cognitive deficit may resemble that encountered in other forms of dementias such as Alzheimer's disease, Parkinson's disease, Pick's disease and vascular dementia.

Treatment and Prognosis

At this time, there is no effective treatment for Huntington's disease. Dopamine blockers such as antipsychotic medications have been reported to be effective in alleviating movement dysfunction when given early in the course of the disease (Folstein, 1989). Such agents are also effective for controlling psychotic symptoms that can occur in the course of the disease. Antidepressants need to be used to treat symptoms of depression. Supportive measures, education, and environmental manipulation may be helpful in dealing with the consequences of cognitive impairment.

The illness is progressive, but is believed to be slower than other primary dementing illnesses. The average duration of the illness is between 13 and 16 years, but some cases may progress over several decades (Lishman, 1987).

8

MENTAL DISORDERS ARISING FROM CEREBROVASCULAR DISEASES

Any serious disruption to the normal circulation of the blood within the brain can lead to major neurological, cognitive, and psychiatric disturbances. Vascular diseases refer mainly to strokes which may be caused by atherosclerotic thrombosis, cerebral embolism, intracranial hemorrhages, and ruptured aneurysms. Other vascular diseases include subarachnoid, subdural and epidural hematomas, and inflammatory diseases of cerebral blood vessels. Psychiatric conditions that can arise from such diseases include dementia, anxiety, depression, mania, psychosis, and personality changes.

VASCULAR (MULTIINFARCT) DEMENTIA

Definition and Clinical Features

Vascular or multiinfarct dementia refers to cognitive impairment that results from cerebrovascular disease.

Unlike Alzheimer's disease in which intellectual impairment is global, cognitive impairment in vascular dementia is usually "patchy" where some intellectual functions may remain relatively intact early in the course of the disease. In addition, focal neurological signs and symptoms are present (DSM-IV, 1994).

The onset is typically abrupt, and the course is erratic and unpredictable. In early stages, cognitive impairments characteristically fluctuate in severity from day to day, and even from hour to hour. Clouding of consciousness develops early and occurs mostly towards the evening. Once the vascular condition is established and settled, neurological and cognitive deficits can be assessed. Cognitive impairment involves memory, abstract thinking, impulse control, and personality (see Chapter 3 and Table 4). The capacity for judgment and a sufficient degree of insight may remain relatively intact for a surprisingly long time. This may cause the patient to react with anxiety and depression regarding his or her cognitive deficits. Emotional lability and a tendency towards outbursts of sudden weeping or laughing may occur (Lishman, 1987).

Neurological symptoms and signs depend on the areas of the brain that are involved in the vascular disorder. Common early symptoms include headache, dizziness, tinnitus, and syncope. Visual disturbances, weaknesses in the extremities, sensory changes, dysphagia (difficulty swallowing), and dysarthria (difficulty speaking) commence soon after. Permanent neurological deficits may later develop. Clinical evidence for vascular disease is often present, and physical examination along with diagnostic investigations may reveal the underlying etiology.

Etiology

Vascular dementia is caused primarily by the accumulation of multiple and repetitive brain infarcts or strokes that can be caused by thromboembolism from extracranial arteries or the heart. It can also develop in association with atherosclerosis of cerebral blood vessels. Hypertension appears to be involved in most cases of vascular dementia. In such instances, small vessel occlusions and hemorrhages develop and lead to small brain infarcts. Other conditions that may contribute to the cerebral vascular disease include diabetes mellitus, collagen vascular diseases, leukemia or polycythemia, rheumatic valvular disease of the heart, atrial fibrillation, and carotid artery stenosis or occlusion (Lishman, 1987).

Differential Diagnosis

Vascular dementia should be differentiated from Alzheimer's disease in which cognitive deterioration is gradual and global, and there is no evidence of cerebrovascular disease. However, it is not unlikely that both vascular dementia and Alzheimer's disease coexist. Other causes of dementia may need to be ruled out through appropriate physical examination and diagnostic investigations.

Treatment and Prognosis

There is no specific treatment for vascular dementia. Hypertension needs to be brought under control, and underlying cerebrovascular disease needs to be treated appropriately to prevent deterioration and further infarction of brain tissue. Psychotropic medications may be used to treat associated symptoms of anxiety, depression, or behavioral changes. Supportive measures and family education are helpful as in all cases of dementias.

Cognitive deficits in the course of vascular dementia are usually stable and may not worsen unless further strokes take place. In such events, deterioration is abrupt and usually follows cerebrovascular accidents. Acute exacerbations may be followed by relative improvement for a time after the vascular event is settled. The course of the disease tends to last longer than Alzheimer's disease, and the final outcome depends on the severity of the underlying vascular disease.

POSTSTROKE DEPRESSION

Definition and Clinical Features

Poststroke depression refers to a depressive disorder that evolves following a stroke. The symptoms are virtually identical to those encountered in "primary" depressive disorders and can be severe enough to meet the diagnostic criteria of major depression.

Robinson, Starr et al. (1983) estimated that between 30% and 50% of patients who suffer acute strokes will develop some form of depressive disorder that is comparable to major depression or dysthymia. In another study, Robinson, Bolduc & Price (1987) found that most patients with severe depression recovered within one to two years following the stroke, while many patients with minor depressive symptoms remained depressed beyond the two years. It has been suggested that the location of brain lesion may influence the duration of depressive symptoms following the stroke. Starkstein and Robinson (1992) reported that patients who suffer from cortical lesions tend to have a slower rate of recovery than those with subcortical and brain stem lesions.

Etiology and Pathophysiology

The exact mechanism of the development of depression following a stroke remains unknown. However, several observations have been reported in that regard. Robinson, Kubos et al. (1984) found that patients with left hemispheric strokes were much more likely to develop depression than those with right hemispheric strokes. They also found that patients with more anterior lesions were more likely to develop depression as compared to patients with posterior lesions.

In addition, it has been suggested that other factors influence the development of poststroke depression, including a premorbid subcortical atrophy and the presence of a family or personal history of mood disorders (Starkstein & Robinson, 1992).

It has been suggested that one of the causes of poststroke depression involves dysfunction of the biogenic amine system, leading to severe depletions of noradrenaline and serotonin as a result of vascular lesions (Robinson, Kubos et al., 1984).

Diagnosis

Depressive symptoms of variable degrees can develop following a stroke. In some patients, the symptoms may meet DSM-IV diagnostic criteria for depression, while in others they may be mild and transient. Cognitive impairment may be present and often makes it difficult to make the proper diagnosis. Other neurological symptoms may also interfere with the clinical picture.

Treatment and Prognosis

Poststroke depression must be treated promptly and aggressively as soon as it is diagnosed. Antidepressant medications are highly effective in that regard. Electroconvulsive therapy has also been used effectively in certain patients. Individual supportive psychotherapy and family therapy are important as well. Rehabilitation of physical, speech, and cognitive impairments needs to be pursued whenever possible.

As indicated above, poststroke depression tends to linger for months and even years. Effective treatment is likely to shorten the course of the depression and improve the general prognosis of the stroke. Starkstein and Robinson (1992) indicated that if depression develops following a stroke the patient's physical recovery tends to be retarded for two years or more.

OTHER PSYCHIATRIC SYMPTOMS ASSOCIATED
WITH STROKES

Poststroke Anxiety

Generalized anxiety disorder is reported to be rare following a stroke. The presence of anxiety was found to be frequently associated with a prior history of alcohol abuse. The incidence of poststroke anxiety, however, is much higher when major depression is also present. Almost 50% of patients with major poststroke depression meet DSM-III diagnostic criteria for generalized anxiety disorder as well (Starkstein & Robinson, 1992).

Treatment of poststroke anxiety disorder is similar to that of generalized anxiety disorder.

Poststroke Mania

Poststroke mania occurs following a stroke involving the right hemisphere in the areas of the cortical or subcortical limbic-related regions. Symptoms include elation, pressured speech, flight of ideas, grandiose thoughts, insomnia, hallucinations, and paranoid delusions. Genetic predisposition to affective disorders and subcortical atrophy may constitute risk factors for poststroke mania (Starkstein & Robinson, 1992).

Poststroke mania can be treated with lithium, anticonvulsant, or antipsychotic medications.

Poststroke Psychosis

Hallucinations and delusions have been reported following strokes. Simple and complex auditory as well as visual hallucinations can occur, depending on the location of the lesion. Visual illusions are also common. Delusions are often related to the hallucinatory experience and may involve elaborate themes. Paranoid or grandiose delusions are also common. High-potency antipsychotic medications may be effective in the treatment of poststroke delusions, yet may be of little help for hallucinatory symptoms (Singer & Read, 1989).

9

PSYCHIATRIC DISORDERS ARISING FROM BRAIN TUMORS

In addition to neurological and physical symptoms, brain tumors are capable of producing a wide variety of psychiatric symptoms that can be difficult to distinguish from those encountered in other psychiatric disorders. The location of the tumor within the brain, along with the type, the size, and the rate of growth of the tumor can influence its neurologic as well as psychiatric manifestations. Depression, mania, hallucinations, delusions, anxiety, delirium, dementia, and personality changes are frequent presentations.

Brain tumors are relatively common, with a prevalence rate of 80 per 100,000 people. It has been estimated that as many as 1%–2% of patients diagnosed with a psychiatric disorder may actually have undiagnosed CNS tumors (Price, Goetz & Lovell, 1992).

FRONTAL LOBE TUMORS

Clinical manifestations of frontal lobe tumors are variable and depend largely on the location of the lesion. Tumors involving the orbitofrontal areas produce disinhibiting symptoms. In such cases, the patient presents with inappropriate social and sexual conduct, emotional lability, euphoria, poor insight and judgment, and distractibility. Tumors involving the frontal convexities are likely to cause symptoms of apathy, indifference, psychomotor retardation, and occasional aggressive outbursts. Tumors involving the medial frontal area usually lead to decrease in spontaneous movement and gestures, mutism, failure to respond to commands, and incontinence (Cummings, 1985).

Psychiatric symptoms that can develop in the course of frontal lobe tumors may include depression, hallucinations, delusions, cognitive deficits, and personality changes. In some cases, these symptoms may precede the onset of neurological signs and symptoms, leading to misdiagnosis and serious delay in providing specific treatment.

TEMPORAL LOBE TUMORS

Tumors of the temporal lobe produce perhaps the highest incidence of mental disturbances (Lishman, 1987). Most symptoms are related to temporal lobe epilepsy that is likely to develop in association with such tumors. These symptoms include paroxysmal rage episodes, hypergraphia, hyperreligiosity, automatism, rapid mood changes, and olfactory, visual, and auditory hallucinations (see Chapter 11).

Other symptoms that are not related to epilepsy (interictal) include schizophrenia-like syndrome manifesting with delusions, hallucinations, and formal thought disorder. In addition, and like frontal lobe tumors, temporal lobe tumors may produce depression, apathy, irritability, and euphoria. Other symptoms include anxiety, panic attacks, cognitive deficits, and personality changes (Price, Goetz & Lovell, 1992).

PARIETAL LOBE TUMORS

Tumors of the parietal lobe are less likely to produce psychiatric symptoms or behavioral changes. However, in some patients, depression and apathy can occur. Cognitive impairment may also develop. In rare cases, paranoid ideation and tactile hallucinations have been reported (Lishman, 1987).

Neurological symptoms of parietal lobe tumors consist of complex and atypical sensory and motor abnormalities which may make the diagnosis more difficult (Price, Goetz & Lovell, 1992).

OCCIPITAL LOBE TUMORS

Tumors of the occipital lobe usually produce visual illusions and hallucinations. In addition, significant cognitive impairment may be seen due to perceptual deficits.

OTHER BRAIN TUMORS

Tumors of the diencephalic region (deep midline areas and close to the limbic system) are likely to produce psychosis, depression, memory disturbances, and personality changes. Tumors near the hypothalamus may cause disorders in eating behavior and hypersomnia. Tumors of the pituitary gland may cause various endocrine disorders, some of which may present with psychiatric symptoms (see Chapter 13).

CLINICAL DIAGNOSIS

Brain tumors typically present with a group of physical and neurological signs and symptoms that often alert the physician to pursue a series of diagnostic investigations which will invariably confirm the diagnosis. However, in some instances, these physical and neurological manifestations may be delayed for unclear reasons and may be preceded by behavioral and psychological symptoms. It is in that population of patients that misdiagnosis can easily occur and treatment may be delayed, with possible serious consequences.   Therefore, it is absolutely essential to pursue a complete diagnostic work-up whenever the index of suspicion is high.

Physical and neurological signs and symptoms are caused by the increase of intracranial pressure that often accompanies brain tumors and by local impact on brain tissue as a result of pressure or erosion by the tumor. Common physical symptoms include headaches, dizziness, nausea and vomiting, and visual disturbances. Neurological symptoms depend on the location of the tumor and may include motor weakness or paralysis, sensory loss, speech problems, ataxia, loss of balance, and seizures. Such clinical presentation is highly suggestive of a brain tumor and should lead the physician to pursue diagnostic measures.

As indicated earlier, in some patients, the initial clinical presentation may be limited to certain behavioral changes and psychiatric symptoms that may point in the direction of primary psychiatric disorders. Brain tumors may present with almost any psychiatric symptom, including psychosis, depression, euphoria, dementia, and personality changes. Therefore, all psychiatric disorders that present with such symptoms need to be considered in the differential diagnosis of brain tumors.

Patients at risk for being misdiagnosed with a "primary" psychiatric disorder in lieu of a brain tumor that is presenting with psychiatric symptoms include those with a relatively sudden onset of psychiatric symptoms in the absence of any past history or family history of psychiatric illness. Such patients usually present with appropriate affect and good insight towards their problems. They often show adequate concern regarding their abnormal behavior and may present with atypical clinical course. Such inconsistent findings should alert the clinician to the possibility of an "organic" etiology. A proper referral should then be made to pursue complete physical, neurological, and mental status examination, along with appropriate diagnostic procedures. Special investigative techniques that can be of diagnostic value include EEG, brain CT scan, and brain MRI. Neuropsychological testing may be helpful in determining the degree of cognitive impairment and the response to treatment.

TREATMENT MODALITIES AND PROGNOSIS

Brain tumors may require various combinations of treatments, including surgery, radiation, and chemotherapy. Responses to treatment may vary depending on the nature and the stage of the tumor. Psychiatric symptoms, including depression, euphoria, anxiety, and psychosis, generally respond favorably to traditional psychotropic medications used in various psychiatric disorders. Patients with brain tumors may be more sensitive to side effects of psychotropic medications such as sedation and anticholinergic and extrapyramidal properties. Lower doses are generally recommended for such patients. In addition, drug-drug interaction potential should be evaluated carefully. Electroconvulsive therapy may be used in selected patients with refractory depression provided that the brain tumor is not associated with increased intracranial pressure (Zwil et al., 1990). Cognitive deficits and personality changes do not respond to medications and may be irreversible in advanced cases.

The prognosis depends mainly on early diagnosis and the success of treatment modalities. While some cases may lead to fatalities, others are curable. In many situations, the patients may be left with motor and sensory deficits. Various types of seizures may develop as a result of the tumor itself or surgical treatment. Antiepileptic medications need to be added in such cases. Psychiatric

symptoms may persist for a long time and may require
ongoing therapy. Individual psychotherapy and family
sessions for support and education can be of great value in
some cases. It is essential to prepare the patient and the
family for the anticipated outcome of the disease and
treatment, which may include permanent disability or
even impending death. Some patients who are completely
cured may continue to be fearful of recurrence and may
experience anxiety and depression for a long time.
Premorbid level of functioning and adaptive capacity will
have a great impact on the total outcome of the treatment.
Finally, cognitive and physical rehabilitation may be
needed and can be highly beneficial in many cases.

10

PSYCHIATRIC MANIFESTATIONS OF TRAUMATIC BRAIN INJURIES

It is estimated that over two million people suffer traumatic brain injuries in the United States each year. Motor vehicle accidents account for approximately one half of traumatic brain injuries. Other causes include falls, assaults, and accidents related to sports and recreation. The total economic cost of traumatic brain injury in the United States is over $25 billion annually. The cost of long-term rehabilitation of each victim may exceed $4 million over a 5–10 year period. Each year, between 70,000 and 90,000 of the survivors are often left with some kind of chronic sequelae due to their original injuries (Department of Health and Human Services, 1989).

Some of the sequelae of traumatic brain injuries may be limited to neurologic deficits, yet most of the disabilities reported are caused by psychological and social impairment. Such disabilities often create a great deal of stress and agony for both the victims and their families. In addition, such injuries often lead to lengthy and controversial legal battles involving victims, employers, insurance companies, and others. The roles of the psychiatrist and the neuropsychologist have become more and more essential in assessing the degree of psychiatric disturbance and cognitive impairment, and determining the prognosis and the degree of permanent disability.

ANATOMY AND NEUROPHYSIOLOGY

Brain injury may be produced by sudden movement of the brain within the skull, as in cases of concussion, by intracranial bleeding as in cases of subarachnoid, subdural, or epidural hemorrhages, or by direct injury to the brain tissue due to penetration by sharp objects such as bullets or bone fragments following car accidents and other industrial injuries. Many cases of concussion, subarachnoid hemorrhage, and subdural hemorrhage may be produced by closed head injury where no skull fracture occurs. On the other hand, epidural hemorrhage often follows severe head injury that leads to skull fracture. Gunshot wounds and injuries caused by other penetrating objects often lead to significant loss of brain tissue, with serious neurological and psychiatric sequelae.

Symptoms may be caused by a variety of pathological processes, including brain edema, brain contusion, pressure by hematomas, brain hypoxia, diffuse axonal injury, loss of brain tissue, and seizures. It has been shown that traumatic brain injury can affect neurotransmitter systems that mediate mood and affect. Neurotransmitters that can be affected include norepinephrine, serotonin, dopamine, and acetylcholine (Silver, Hales & Yudofsky, 1992).

CLINICAL FEATURES

Traumatic brain injuries often lead to a combination of neurologic and psychiatric manifestations. Some of these manifestations occur soon after the accident, while others develop slowly and gradually over weeks and months. The clinical picture depends largely on the nature and extent of the injury, and on the parts of the brain that have been most affected by the injury.

I. Early Manifestations

These features are generally seen immediately following the injury, or soon after gaining consciousness.

A. Loss of Consciousness

Loss of consciousness can follow any type of traumatic brain injury, from concussion to severe skull fractures. The onset is almost immediate following the injury, and may last from few moments, as in cases of concussion, to several weeks or months as seen in cases of coma. Periods of unconsciousness lasting for more than a few hours may be associated with permanent brain damage and long term mental sequelae (Lishman, 1987).

B. Delirium and Psychosis

As the patient with brain injury gains consciousness, symptoms of delirium may be observed, including disorientation, clouding of consciousness, restlessness, and agitation. Hallucinations and delusions may be encountered. The duration of the confusional state depends on the severity of the injury and the length of the period of unconsciousness. A patient who sustains a momentary concussion may return to a normal state within a few minutes, while another who lapses into a deep coma for several hours may take several days or weeks before returning to normal.

C. Amnesia

Most patients, upon sustaining a period of unconsciousness, may suffer from loss of memory of the events surrounding the accident and those immediately preceding the injury, a phenomenon known as "retrograde amnesia." This type of amnesia usually involves the loss of memory for minutes, hours, or days preceding the injury.

Some of the lost memory may be recovered as the patient recovers from the acute effects of the head injury. On the other hand, amnesia may involve some events that occur after the injury (during and after recovering from unconsciousness). These events may fail to be recorded in memory for a period of time, leading to what is known as "posttraumatic amnesia." In such cases, the amnesia may last from several minutes to several weeks and finally ends sharply with the return of normal continuous memory.

As indicated earlier, retrograde amnesia is generally shorter than posttraumatic amnesia. It has been noted that posttraumatic amnesia is likely to be prolonged in more severe cases of brain injury. Furthermore, it has been demonstrated that prolonged posttraumatic amnesia is more likely to be followed by more severe psychiatric disabilities and intellectual impairment (Lishman, 1987).

II. Delayed Manifestations

These features are usually noted weeks or months following the trauma. The extent of such sequelae is dependent on several factors, including the severity of the brain injury, the location of brain lesion, premorbid personality and psychological profile, and history of alcohol abuse. Patients with premorbid personality traits and preexisting psychiatric conditions are more likely to report serious psychiatric and cognitive impairment following traumatic brian injuries. Furthermore, it has been reported (Ruff et al., 1990) that victims of traumatic brain injury who had a history of alcohol abuse had more severe sequelae as compared to patients without such a history.

A. Personality Changes

Most of the changes in personality and behavior following traumatic brain injury represent the exacerbation and accentuation of preexisting personality traits such as disorderliness, suspiciousness, and anxiousness. It appears that the injury leads to a certain degree of disinhibition, irritability, and lack of tolerance that causes the patient to act in ways that are socially inappropriate or to exhibit anger and aggressive behavior more readily. Social withdrawal, apathy, inappropriate sexual behavior, and lack of attention to personal hygiene are common manifestations. Some patients are aware of the changes that have occurred and may show adequate concern, while others are unaware of the changes and may become defensive and belligerent when confronted. Kreutzer and Zasler (1989) studied the changes in sexual behavior in male patients following brain injury. They found that most victims had decreased sex drive, erectile problems, and diminished frequency of intercourse. Female victims report decreased sex drive as well. Personality changes tend to occur rather suddenly following the injury and may last for many years and even become permanent.

B. Cognitive Deficits

Cognitive deficits vary depending on the location of the injury and on its severity. Injuries due to penetrating objects and depressed skull fractures often cause focal cognitive deficits that may become permanent. On the other hand, closed head injuries and concussions tend to cause generalized intellectual impairment of variable degrees. Such deficits usually recover fully within weeks or months, but subtle changes that are too minor to detect may persist. In certain patients with relatively mild head injuries, significant cognitive deficits may persist for many years despite the lack of brain damage or any physical evidence to support the complaints (Lishman, 1987).

Most intellectual aspects affected by head injury involve mental sluggishness, poor memory, poor concentration, diminished abstraction ability, poor calculation, and reduced ability to process information, reason, and plan. Children who survive head injury often develop learning disabilities and behavioral problems. This becomes evident when neuropsychological testing is carried out or when the child returns to school (Silver et al., 1992).

C. Psychiatric Manifestations

Among psychiatric symptoms that can follow traumatic brain injury, depression takes the lead. Varney, Hartzke, and Roberts (1987) studied patients after closed head injury and found that 77% of these patients met DSM-III diagnostic criteria for major depression. They added that 46% of the depressed patients experienced their symptoms six months after the injury. Apathy, sadness, and grief reactions are common. Although major depression can develop, the clinical presentation may not be typical. Suicidal ideation and attempts are common even years after the injury.

It is important to carefully evaluate the patient to determine whether or not depressive symptoms preceded the accident or occurred thereafter. The severity of depression is usually not related to the duration of loss of consciousness, the duration of posttraumatic amnesia, or the presence or absence of skull fracture. Rather, it was found to be mostly related to the extent of neuropsychological impairment (Silver et al., 1992).

Psychotic symptoms are also common after traumatic brain injury. Early psychotic symptoms are usually due to delirium and often resolve in a relatively short time. However, delayed psychotic symptoms can occur in a clear state of consciousness, and can simulate schizophrenia, including symptoms of hallucinations and paranoid delusions.

Most patients who sustain traumatic brain injury are described as tense or anxious. Symptoms of anxiety can last for years after the injury. In addition, such patients are at risk of developing posttraumatic stress disorder (PTSD). In rare instances, cases of obsessive compulsive disorder have also been reported subsequent to traumatic brain injury (Silver et al., 1992).

D. Aggressive Behavior

The majority of victims of traumatic brain injury suffer from irritability and aggressive behavior that can last for years following the trauma (McKinlay et al, 1981). Such behavior is often reported by families of patients, since spouses and other close family members become the subject of such violence. Aggressive behavior can result from focal or diffuse brain lesions involving various cortical and subcortical brain tissue. Some of the cases may be due to epileptic phenomena, while others are caused by disinhibition and dyscontrol. The behavior may be persistent or episodic and is not always triggered by precipitating factors. This form of disability often requires ongoing psychiatric management of the patient and supportive work for the family.

E. Postconcussion Syndrome

This condition refers to certain somatic, perceptual, cognitive, and emotional symptoms that develop and may persist following minor brain injuries. Minor brain injury is typically associated with a brief period of unconsciousness (less than 20 minutes) or no loss of consciousness, and no physical evidence of brain damage. Most of these patients do not require hospitalization, yet they continue to report various symptoms that can persist for years. The symptoms include headache, dizziness, fatigue, insomnia, poor memory, impaired concentration, sensitivity to noise or light, depression, anxiety, and irritability. Most of these symptoms cannot be explained based on the brain injury; all diagnostic tests, including brain imaging studies, are often normal. In general, postconcussion syndrome should improve within three months. However, some patients continue to report residual symptoms for years. Posttraumatic stress disorder (PTSD) can also complicate the condition (Silver et al., 1992).

This syndrome remains controversial among researchers and clinicians. Some authors believe that it can be associated with diffuse axonal damage of neurons, while others believe that it is purely "functional." Preexisting personality organization, past psychiatric history, and the prospects of compensation and litigation may play a role in the persistence of the syndrome.

F. Epilepsy

Various forms of epilepsy can result from traumatic brain injuries, especially the penetrating type or those associated with depressed skull fracture. Temporal lobe epilepsy involves a group of psychiatric and behavioral manifestations that can add to the complications of traumatic brain injury. Epileptic disorders are discussed in detail in Chapter Eleven.

DIAGNOSIS AND FOLLOW-UP STUDIES

Victims of traumatic brain injuries are often taken to emergency rooms for immediate medical attention. Patients require complete physical and neurological examinations to determine the extent of the injury and its impact on various brain and body functions. Diagnostic procedures include CT scan of the head and of other areas as indicated. MRI of the brain may be needed in many situations to assess the degree of brain damage, especially when CT scan fails to show any brain lesions to correlate with the neuropsychiatric consequences of the injury. Electroencephalography can be helpful in detecting seizure activity or other abnormalities resulting from the trauma.

As the medical condition is stabilized, the psychiatrist may be consulted to assist in the diagnosis and management of various psychiatric manifestations, including delirium, psychosis, depression, anxiety, personality changes, and cognitive deficits. Complete psychiatric history and a thorough mental status examination are essential steps to establish a baseline of psychopathology after the accident. Symptom rating scales that rate behavior, amnesia, cognition, depression, and aggression may be helpful in establishing baseline deficits. Frequent and periodic assessments may be needed to monitor the patient's progress. Neuropsychological testing is often needed, especially in cases that seem to take a chronic course.

Such testing may be essential to document cognitive and intellectual deficits and may provide important information that pertains to the location and severity of brain damage. Neuropsychological testing may be repeated every six month to a year to evaluate progress and assign disability.

It is essential that the clinician evaluate premorbid personality traits along with any other pertinent psychiatric history to assess the effect of such factors on the outcome of traumatic brain injury. In certain susceptible individuals, it is not uncommon that head injury might precipitate a serious psychiatric disorder such as schizophrenia or major depression, or the injury might enhance preexisting personality traits and turn them into a disorder. In such examples, the brain injury serves as a catalyst that accelerates the onset of a condition that would have presented itself later or under other circumstances. It is also essential that the psychiatrist evaluate patients for potential malingering for the purpose of litigation and secondary gain.

TREATMENT MODALITIES

The treatment of victims of traumatic brain injury involves the cooperation and coordination of various medical specialists and support staff. Some patients with mild head injury may not be admitted to the hospital and may be seen by a neurologist for follow-up. Patients with penetrating injuries and skull fractures require immediate medical care that is usually provided by the neurosurgeon, the neurologist, and other medical specialists as needed. The psychiatrist often joins the team to manage psychiatric and behavioral problems.

Psychiatric disorders are treated independently as in nontraumatic conditions. Delirium and psychosis often respond to mild sedation with a high-potency antipsychotic agent. Depression is treated with antidepressant medications and manic episodes may be managed with lithium or anticonvulsant agents. Anxiety and panic attacks are managed with benzodiazepines, buspirone or antidepressants. Insomnia may resolve spontaneously as the neurological and psychiatric disorders resolve. If needed, short-acting benzodiazepines may be prescribed for a brief period of time. Alcohol, barbiturates, and long-acting benzodiazepines should be avoided.

As a rule, patients with traumatic brain injury are highly sensitive to sedating agents and are more susceptible to side effects. It is always important to bear in mind that most antidepressant and antipsychotic medications are capable of lowering the seizure threshold; hence, they may introduce further complications into the already complicated situation. Therefore, these agents should be used with caution. Lower doses should be introduced initially and increased as tolerated. The agent should be selected based on the side-effect profile that is least likely to complicate the clinical condition.

Personality changes do not respond to medication treatment. Behavioral therapy, environmental interventions, and family therapy may be helpful. Aggressive behavior and violent episodes may be treated with various psychotropic agents, including antipsychotics, antidepressants, benzodiazepines, buspirone, lithium, anticonvulsants, and beta blockers. Cognitive deficits may improve spontaneously; however, cognitive rehabilitation may offer an opportunity for faster and a more complete recovery. Stimulants such as Ritalin may be used for apathy, poor attention, and impaired concentration. However, such agents may increase the patient's irritability and can cause depression if withdrawn abruptly.

Finally, individual psychotherapy for support and education is often needed to help the patient cope with his or her deficit and return to work and normal life as soon as possible. The spouse and other family members often need to be involved in the treatment so that the benefits of psychotherapy may be maximized.

PROGNOSIS AND MEDICOLEGAL CONSIDERATIONS

Most cases of traumatic brain injury recover with little or no sequelae. However, regardless of the severity of the original injury, a group of patients continues to report psychiatric symptoms and cognitive deficits months or years after the accident. In cases where physical brain damage or loss has occurred, it is possible to predict the prognosis with some degree of certainty. However, in cases where no brain damage could be detected, it is much more difficult to make an accurate prognosis. Patients with postconcussion syndrome tend to represent the majority of those patients who continue to report psychiatric and cognitive deficits. While neuropsychological testing can be of help in such cases, it may not be able to pick out all malingerers and patients with exaggerated self-report.

The question of prognosis and permanent psychiatric disability is always asked by attorneys in cases involving litigation and worker's compensation. The clinician must be totally objective in his or her opinion of the nature of the disability regardless of the legal issues involved. Repeated examinations and neuropsychological testing every six months can give the clinician some sense of whether or not the patient is making any progress. As long as the patient continues to show progress, no final prognosis should be given. In cases where the clinical condition does not change over a year, a final prognosis may be given. The clinician should feel comfortable telling the court that he or she is unable to give a definite prognosis or assign permanent disability due to the unpredictable nature of the condition.

11

PSYCHIATRIC ASPECTS
OF SEIZURE DISORDERS

Although epilepsy is no longer classified with mental disorders, a strong link has existed between seizures and psychiatry for at least a century. It has been estimated that about 20% of epileptic outpatients suffer from some kind of significant psychopathology. The incidence of psychosis among epileptic patients is about 7%, which is significantly higher than that among nonepileptic individuals. Conversely, the prevalence of epilepsy among patients in psychiatric hospitals is 2%–3% as compared to the general population where the prevalence is 1.5%. These figures suggest that patients with seizure disorders are at a much greater risk of developing psychiatric and behavioral problems, especially psychoses (Neppe & Tucker, 1992).

Seizures result from abnormal electrical discharges of brain neurons that can lead to a series of clinical phenomena involving neurological and psychiatric symptoms. Neurological symptoms include loss or alteration of consciousness, disorientation, amnesia, and sensory or motor disturbances. Psychiatric and behavioral symptoms include psychosis, depression, anxiety, agitation, cognitive disturbances, and personality changes.

CLASSIFICATION

Seizure disorders may be classified as partial seizures or generalized seizures. Partial seizures represent focal or localized activity involving simple motor, sensory, or autonomic manifestations without changes in the level of consciousness. Complex partial seizures (temporal lobe epilepsy) almost always lead to changes in the level of consciousness along with stereotyped movements and several behavioral and psychiatric symptoms. Partial seizure can evolve into generalized seizures and may then be classified as such. Generalized seizures often involve impairment of consciousness and consist of episodes of absences (petit mal), myoclonic seizures, or tonic-clonic seizures (grand mal) (Alexopoulos, 1989).

CLINICAL MANIFESTATIONS

Several behavioral changes can be observed in patients with epilepsy. The onset can take place before, during, or after the seizure.

Preictal (Before-the-Seizure/Prodromal) Symptoms

These events occur immediately before the onset of the seizure itself. They can last for a variable period of time, ranging from a few minutes to several days. The symptoms include personality changes, irritability, clouded thinking, poor concentration, and mood lability. Occasionally, overt psychotic symptoms may develop. Preictal events are more common in children and in patients with complex partial seizures. Most of these symptoms disappear after the onset of the seizure (Alexopoulos, 1989; Neppe & Tucker, 1992).

Ictal (During-the-Seizure) Symptoms

Ictal phenomena begin with the epileptic aura, which may last for a few seconds to one minute. The clinical manifestations of auras range from simple sensations to complex behavioral and ideational disturbances. Following that, the seizure occurs; it may be focal or generalized. The symptoms that occur during the seizure correlate to a large extent with the areas of the brain in which the seizure originates (Alexopoulos, 1989). Most common psychiatric symptoms that occur as part of the ictal events include automatism, behavioral aberrations, cognitive changes, altered consciousness, derealization, depersonalization, and paranoid ideation (Neppe & Tucker, 1992).

Complex Partial Seizures (Temporal Lobe Epilepsy)

Complex partial seizures or TLE, which is also known as psychomotor epilepsy, represent a series of behavioral and psychiatric symptoms that can vary widely and mimic almost any psychiatric disorder. Symptoms include sudden onset of automatic movement of the lips, altered level of consciousness, forced thinking, hypergraphia (excessive writing), hypersexuality, and hyperreligiosity. Certain patients present with episodes of uncontrollable rage and violence that are usually aimless and not directed at specific people or things, and is followed by amnesia of the episode. More elaborate clinical presentations may involve psychotic symptomatology, including various forms of olfactory, gustatory, visual, and auditory hallucinations. Other psychiatric symptoms include depression and profound mood changes with fear and anxiety. Illusions, flashbacks, and déjà vu phenomena often occur. Some patients enter fugue states and wander for hours or days, appearing perplexed, disoriented, and incoherent.

Postictal (After-the-Seizure) Symptoms

After the seizure is concluded, patients may feel drowsy or sleep for a short period of time. Some patients become disoriented, agitated, or paranoid. Visual and auditory hallucinations and intense mood changes can occur during this phase.

Psychiatric Manifestations of Interictal (Between-the-Seizures) Periods

As indicated earlier, the incidence of psychiatric disorders among patients with seizure disorders is significantly higher than in the general population. This is particularly true for patients with complex partial seizures. Psychiatric disorders include psychosis, anxiety, mood disorders, personality disorders, and cognitive impairment (Pond & Bidwell, 1960).

Psychosis in epileptic patients often resembles schizophrenia and is referred to as schizophreniform disorder. Symptoms include mild cognitive impairment, unfixed delusions, systematized paranoid delusions, various forms of hallucinations, and manic-like symptoms (Neppe & Tucker, 1992).

Depression and anxiety in the epileptic population are also common. Various degrees of severity have been observed by different researchers. It has been reported (Barraclough, 1981) that epileptic patients have a five times higher risk of suicide as compared to the general population.

Personality profile of the epileptic patient has been somewhat controversial. Some authors describe epileptic patients as argumentative, persistent, suspicious, irritable, circumstantial, and egocentric (Alexopoulos, 1989). These traits have not been observed by other researchers in the majority of patients, although a small number of patients seem to present with such traits (Pond & Bidwell, 1960).

Cognitive disturbances are common in patients with epilepsy, especially in those with partial seizures with a focus at the temporal lobe. The deficits include impairment in attention, concentration, memory, and verbal abilities. Cognitive deficits are less frequent in patients with tonic-clonic seizures and rarely occur in patients with petit mal. In general, patients with seizure disorders have lower intelligence scores as compared to the general population (Alexopoulos, 1989).

ETIOLOGY AND PATHOPHYSIOLOGY

Seizure disorders can be caused by a wide variety of pathological processes affecting the brain. Causes include head trauma, brain tumors, meningitis and encephalitis, endocrine and metabolic diseases, drug side effects and withdrawal states, and genetic predisposition. Cases of unspecified etiology are labeled as "idiopathic." The behavioral and psychological manifestations of seizures are probably caused by chronic electrical discharges or chemical changes in various areas of the brain. It is likely that psychiatric symptoms are caused by alterations in various neurotransmitter systems, including dopamine, serotonin, norepinephrine, and others, as a result of the pathological process responsible for the seizure.

It has been suggested that the location of the epileptogenic focus may determine the nature of the psychiatric symptomatology. Trimble (1984) reported that epileptic patients who develop psychosis have the epileptogenic focus in the dominant hemisphere more frequently than patients without psychotic symptoms. Flor-Henry (1969) suggested that epileptic patients who present with mood disorders frequently have the epileptogenic focus in the nondominant hemisphere. Furthermore, it has been suggested that patients with epileptogenic focus in the temporal lobe have a higher incidence of suicide attempts and completed suicides as compared to other epileptic patients (Alexopoulos, 1989). Cognitive disturbances that are observed in some epileptic patients have been explained on the basis of structural brain damage that is responsible for the onset of the seizure disorder. Patients with epileptogenic locus on the dominant side may experience greater impairment in verbal skills, while patients with epileptogenic locus on the nondominant side show greater impairment in nonverbal performance tasks.

DIAGNOSIS AND DIFFERENTIAL DIAGNOSIS

Epilepsy is diagnosed on the basis of clinical evidence and electroencephalographic (EEG) tracing of seizure activity. On some occasions, the EEG may not show any signs for epilepsy despite strong clinical evidence. In such instances, repeated EEGs, sleep EEG, sleep-deprived EEG, extended EEG (12 hours–2 weeks), and special techniques such as nasopharyngeal and sphenoidal electrodes may yield greater chances of positive results. Videotaping patients to observe their behavior during the seizure may offer some clues to the diagnostic question. Recent techniques of brain mapping based on computerized EEG may be useful, especially in cases with psychiatric symptomatology.

Since seizure disorders may present with various psychiatric symptoms, several psychiatric disorders need to be differentiated from seizure disorders. They include schizophreniform disorders, depression, anxiety, dementia, and personality disorders. Careful past history, family history, and EEG examinations may be helpful in that regard.

Other conditions that may be difficult to differentiate from seizure disorders include conversion disorders, dissociative disorders, factitious disorders, and malingering. In all of these conditions, no physical etiology could be found to explain the clinical picture that may resemble true seizures to a great extent. These conditions may be referred to as pseudoseizures, psychogenic, or hysterical seizures. These attacks are often motivated by secondary gain or unconscious factors and are frequently triggered by stress. The movements are usually atypical or purposeful and the fall seldom results in injury. The consciousness is usually preserved and there are no postictal features. EEG recordings are always normal, even when taken during the attack. Unlike some true seizure disorders, pseudoseizures do not result in elevation of prolactin level 20 to 30 minutes after the seizure.

It is essential to emphasize here that epileptic patients who present with psychiatric symptoms should receive complete psychiatric evaluations with detailed history and mental status examination to differentiate various diagnostic possibilities. Occasionally, psychometric assessments, including MMPI, projective testing, and neuropsychological testing, may be needed to evaluate psychological profile and cognitive abilities. These evaluations may be important for making recommendations for social and vocational rehabilitation.

TREATMENT AND PROGNOSIS

Seizure disorders are treated with various anticonvulsants. These include phenytoin, phenobarbital, primidone, carbamazepine, ethosuximide, valproate, clonazepam, and diazepam. These medications can be used individually or in various combinations to control the seizures.

Psychiatric and behavioral symptoms usually respond favorably to the effect of anticonvulsants. However, the additional use of various psychotropic medications may be indicated in certain situations. Antipsychotic agents may be used to control psychotic symptoms or severe agitation. Similarly, antidepressant medications are quite effective for the treatment of depression in the context of seizure disorders. It should be kept in mind, however, that both antipsychotics and antidepressants are capable of lowering the seizure threshold, thus prompting the need for further adjustment of the dosage of anticonvulsant agents. In addition, lithium, beta blockers, buspirone, and benzodiazepines may be used as indicated, depending on the clinical presentation.

Special attention should be paid to the potential occurrence of drug-drug interaction in which blood levels of certain agents may be increased or decreased leading to toxic side effects or reemergence of symptoms. Furthermore, many epileptic patients suffer from psychiatric disorders independent of the seizure disorders. In such instances, traditional psychiatric management is pursued in conjunction with appropriate antiseizure medications.

In addition to pharmacological treatment, various types of psychotherapy may be indicated and can be of significant help to the patient and his or her family. Behavioral modification and biofeedback may also be useful.

PSYCHOSOCIAL ASPECTS OF SEIZURE DISORDERS

Like psychiatric patients, epileptic patients continue to be stigmatized by their illness, causing them serious social and psychological distress. Such individuals are forced to accept the fact that they have a chronic illness that may interfere with their work and life in general, and that they may have to receive medication and be monitored for a long time, perhaps for life. Patients have particular concerns about swimming alone or driving a vehicle. In fact, in many states certain restrictions apply to patients with epilepsy with regard to driving. These restrictions create a new problem for the epileptic patient who may have to become dependent on others. Jobs that require climbing ladders or operating dangerous machinery are not permitted for that population. Many individuals have particular concerns about performing normal social activities, such as dating or being with friends, for fear of being observed during an epileptic seizure.

While many of these fears and restrictions are unnecessary, the reality is that epileptic patients are always subject to a higher degree of risk and are likely to be discriminated against. These factors alone, and regardless of the symptoms caused by the seizure disorder itself, are likely to create many psychological problems for the individual.

Most patients become isolated and avoid social situations. Others become depressed and anxious. It is common to observe personality change in that population, resulting from either the seizure disorder itself or from the reaction and the failure to adapt to the illness. With advances in medical technology and the introduction of new drugs, the management and control of seizure disorders are becoming more successful, allowing patients to lead as normal lives as possible.

12

PSYCHIATRIC MANIFESTATIONS OF CENTRAL NERVOUS SYSTEM INFECTIONS

Infections that involve the brain or the meningeal membranes are capable of producing a wide variety of behavioral, cognitive, and psychological symptoms. Although in most cases such symptoms are limited to irritability, restlessness, and insomnia, in many other instances more serious psychiatric conditions may develop. These include delirium, psychosis, anxiety, mood disorders, dementia, and personality changes. Physical and neurological signs and symptoms are observed, depending on the nature and extent of the infection.

ETIOLOGY AND PATHOPHYSIOLOGY

Infections occurring within the central nervous system may involve the brain itself, meningeal membranes or both. Such infections can be caused by a wide variety of microorganisms. These include viruses, bacteria, fungi, spirochetes, rickettsiae, and parasites. Examples are outlined in Table 9.

TABLE 9
EXAMPLES OF CENTRAL NERVOUS SYSTEM
INFECTIONS

A. VIRAL INFECTIONS:
1. Acquired Immune Deficiency Syndrome (AIDS)
2. Herpes Simplex encephalitis
3. Mumps meningoencephalitis
4. Creutzfeldt-Jakob disease

B. BACTERIAL INFECTIONS:
1. Tuberculous meningitis
2. Meningococcal meningitis
3. Pneumococcal meningitis

C. FUNGAL INFECTIONS:
1. Cryptococcal meningitis
2. Coccidioidal meningitis
3. Candida Albicans meningitis

D. SPIROCHETAL INFECTIONS:
1. Neurosyphilis
2. Lyme Disease

E. RICKETTSIAL INFECTIONS:
1. Rocky Mountain Spotted Fever

F. PROTOZOAL INFECTIONS:
1. Toxoplasmosis
2. Trypanosomiasis
3. Primary amebic meningoencephalitis

Neurological and psychiatric symptoms arise from local pathological changes that occur in brain and meningeal tissues due to inflammatory process. These histological and physiological changes are likely to produce different abnormalities in neurotransmitter systems. This, in turn, may lead to the onset of various behavioral and psychological manifestations that may persist until the inflammatory process is resolved. In chronic conditions, or when irreversible changes such as scarring have occurred in the meninges or brain tissue, residual symptoms may persist indefinitely.

Occasionally, psychiatric symptoms can develop due to systemic infections that originate in organs that are distant from the brain, yet still affect the functions of the brain indirectly due to high fever, hypoxia, or toxins liberated by the infection. Examples include delirium that develops in the course of pneumonia, viral hepatitis, and malaria (see Chapter Two). It is important to note here that severe systemic infections can lead to septicemia where viruses, bacteria, and other microorganisms are disseminated through the blood to other organs, including the brain, where local infections and abscesses can develop.

CLINICAL PRESENTATIONS

I. Acquired Immune Deficiency Syndrome (AIDS)

Since the explosion of the AIDS epidemic in the 1980s, a lot has been learned about the disease and its impact on various organs. The virus responsible for this disease (HIV) has been found to attack the central nervous system in addition to the immune system (Price et al., 1988). While it is rather unlikely that the disease may present initially with psychiatric symptomatology, several cases of AIDS have been reported where psychiatric symptoms preceded other physical signs and symptoms (Marotta & Perry, 1989). Navia, Jordan and Price (1986) reported that 7% of AIDS patients in their study presented with an "organic" psychosis as the initial manifestation of the illness. They added that 16% of all the patients exhibited various psychotic symptoms later on as their condition deteriorated. In many cases the onset of psychiatric symptoms is largely due to the involvement of brain tissue itself with the virus which causes several histological and physiological changes. In others, psychiatric manifestations occur simply due to indirect effects on the brain because of systemic infections and other complications, or because of treatment of HIV with various agents.

Psychiatric manifestations vary considerably from one patient to another, and may mimic to a large extent "primary" psychiatric disorders. Early manifestations may be limited to mental slowing, forgetfulness, apathy, lethargy, social withdrawal, and personality change. In some patients, acute mental status changes occur with typical symptoms of delirium, including disorientation, clouded sensorium, agitation, and extreme irritability. Psychotic symptoms consisting of illusions, hallucination and delusions have been reported as well. Depressive symptoms that resembled "primary" depression were also reported. Mania and other psychiatric symptoms have been observed in certain patients. Chronic mental status changes can develop in certain patients with AIDS. Significant cognitive impairment involving various intellectual abilities occurs after several years of being infected with the virus. Such conditions may be known as AIDS dementia. Along similar lines, personality changes may develop, with serious impairment in social and vocational functions, mood changes, and poor impulse control (Markowitz & Perry, 1992).

Patients who learn that they have been infected with HIV react in many different ways depending on their psychological make-up and their premorbid personality organization. Some patients react with denial where they show very little affect and minimize the seriousness of their problems. Others exhibit severe anxiety and fear. Anger and violent behavior are also common. Most patients react with some degree of depression, especially towards final stages. All reactive psychiatric symptoms should be recognized as such and should be differentiated from those caused by the infection itself.

AIDS phobia represents another psychological condition that arises in certain healthy individuals who may have had some form of contact with patients with AIDS. Fear of "catching" the disease can reach a severe degree leading to obsessional preoccupation or even delusional thinking. This is particularly common in nurses and other medical personnel who may be stuck accidentally with infected needles. Regular blood testing, education, and supportive psychotherapy may be needed for such individuals. However, certain individuals may experience severe AIDS phobia that is not based on any realistic risk or medical facts. In such instances, it is important to search for other sources of psychopathology that may account for the symptoms.

II. Encephalitis and Meningitis

Infection of brain tissue (encephalitis) or surrounding membranes (meningitis) can be caused by a wide variety of viruses, bacteria, and other microorganisms, as outlined in Table 9. Early physical and neurological signs and symptoms consist of malaise, irritability, headache, vomiting, photophobia, fever, and neck rigidity. As the illness progresses, clouded consciousness and focal neurological signs appear. Later, stupor and coma may develop. The progression of the condition can be rapid over days or slow over weeks, depending on the causative agent and the patient's age and general condition. Such infections often occur as complications to respiratory tract infections or ear infections or as a result of septicemia arising from infections in other organs.

These conditions are regarded as serious and can be fatal, especially when treatment may not be available, as in viral encephalitis. Furthermore, such infections, even when resolved, can leave behind neurological sequelae such as sensory or motor impairment, visual or auditory impairment, epilepsy, or parkinsonism.

Psychiatric symptoms may develop during the course of encephalitis or meningitis. They usually accompany neurological and physical signs and symptoms. Occasionally, they may occur alone or dominate the clinical picture, leading to misdiagnosis. Misra and Hay (1971) reported three cases of patients who were admitted to the psychiatric unit with a provisional diagnosis of schizophrenia. Those patients were later found to have encephalitis and were treated accordingly. Wilson (1976) and Crow (1978) presented other striking cases of encephalitis mimicking psychiatric disorders. During the acute phase of encephalitis or meningitis, symptoms of delirium are observed. These include agitation, hallucinations, especially of the visual modality, illusions, and delusions.

After the resolution of the acute phase of these infections, other psychiatric complications may develop. These include depression, hypomania, psychosis, cognitive impairment, and personality changes. Children are particularly at risk for developing behavioral and personality changes following encephalitis. Symptoms included extreme distractibility, restlessness, lack of impulse control, and poor social adjustment (Lishman, 1987).

III. Creutzfeldt-Jakob Disease

This is a very rare dementing disease caused by a slow virus that attacks the brain and other organs. While this disease is not easily transmissible, it has been shown to occur in clusters and to be transmitted among family members. Family history has been reported in 15% of cases studied. It has also been reported to be transmitted via contaminated surgical tools and other equipment (Masters et al., 1979). The disease most commonly strikes people between their 40s and 60s and seems to occur in men as often as in women. The virus attacks cortical and subcortical areas, leading to profound degeneration.

Prodromal symptoms last for weeks or months and consist of fatigue, insomnia, anxiety, depression or elation, mental slowness, and unpredictable behavior. Later, neurological signs such as ataxia, paralysis, rigidity, or tremor develop. Disturbance of speech or vision may occur. Progressive dementia represents a major complication of the disease, with severe cognitive impairment and personality changes. Other psychiatric symptoms include frank delirium, hallucinations, delusions, and depression. The course of the disease is very rapid, and patients usually die within nine months to two years from the time of the onset of the symptoms. Death is usually preceded by deep coma which may last for several weeks (Lishman, 1987).

The illness can be differentiated from Alzheimer's disease and other dementias by its rapid course and the presence of neurological signs. CT scan of the brain may reveal marked cortical atrophy. EEG recordings show consistent abnormalities. It is important to emphasize that in some rare cases Creutzfeldt-Jakob disease may overlap with Alzheimer's disease, leading to a mixed and confusing clinical picture. No treatment is available. However, psychotropic medications and supportive measures may be provided as needed.

IV. Tertiary Syphilis

Syphilitic infections have shown significant decline during the past few decades. This is mostly due to public education and the introduction of penicillin. Nevertheless, in rare cases where the infection may occur, the central nervous system may be involved, leading to what is known as neurosyphilis which presents with several neurological and psychiatric manifestations. Varieties of neurosyphilis include meningovascular syphilis, Tabes Dorsalis, and General Paralysis of the Insane. Meningovascular syphilis and Tabes Dorsalis present mainly with neurological signs and symptoms that are beyond the scope of this book.

General Paralysis of the Insane, also known as Dementia Paralytica, may present with a complicated picture that contains several psychiatric symptoms. The onset is insidious, leading to lethargy, insomnia, memory disturbances, increased irritability, and outbursts of temper. This is followed by impairment of judgment and inappropriate social conduct. Other signs of dementia soon follow. Psychosis in this illness consists mainly of euphoria and grandiose delusions. Paranoid ideation and depression can also occur. Neurological signs include tremor, slurred speech, reflex abnormalities, ataxia, cranial nerve palsy, and other focal neurological signs. Convulsions and strokes may occur. Paresis occur in about 5% of patients.

The disease can be easily diagnosed by serological and other laboratory tests and should be differentiated from manic depressive illness, schizophrenia, and other types of dementia. The illness can be treated effectively with penicillin, but residual brain damage may persist.

V. Lyme Disease

Lyme disease has been rapidly increasing in certain areas of the United States. The spirochete responsible for the illness has been reported to infect brain tissue and lead to various neuropsychiatric manifestations. Kaplan et al. (1992) reported the occurrence of memory impairment, sleep disturbances, and depression in patients with Lyme encephalopathy. Roelcke et al. (1992) reported a case of untreated Lyme disease with neuroborreliosis (CNS infection with Borrelia spirochete) which evolved into acute schizophrenia-like psychosis. More recently, symptoms of major depression, mania, and panic attacks have been reported in patients with Lyme disease. These symptoms remitted after adequate antibiotic treatment (Fallon et al., 1993).

VI. Cerebral Abscess

Cerebral abscesses often occur as a result of extension of infections from the middle ear, mastoid cells, or sinuses. In addition, blood-borne microorganisms of various types originating in distant organs may reach the brain and form cerebral abscesses. Neurological and psychiatric symptoms may arise depending on the size and the location of the abscess. For all practical purposes, clinical presentation of cerebral abscess is very much like that of cerebral tumors (see Chapter Nine). The condition can be diagnosed with CT scans and should be differentiated from brain tumors. Treatment may require surgical intervention to drain the abscess, along with antibiotic therapy.

DIAGNOSIS AND DIFFERENTIAL DIAGNOSIS

Correct diagnosis of intracranial infections is highly important due to the seriousness of the condition. Most of these patients are seen first by their family physician and other specialists who manage the medical condition as needed. The psychiatrist may be called later as behavioral and psychiatric symptoms emerge. In rare instances, such patients may present initially with psychiatric symptoms and may be seen first by mental health professionals. Whenever the clinician has any suspicion that the symptoms may be caused by a medical condition, the patient must be referred to appropriate specialists as soon as possible. Diagnostic procedures include detailed physical and neurological examination, mini-mental status examination, complete battery of blood tests, lumbar puncture, cultures, EEG, CT scan and MRI of the brain, and other tests as needed.

Psychiatric symptoms presenting in the course of encephalitis or meningitis should be differentiated from "primary" psychiatric disorders such as schizophrenia, mania, depression, dementia, and personality disorders. Careful past history along with proper medical investigations are likely to resolve the uncertainties. Mental disorders due to other medical conditions may resemble those resulting from meningoencephalitis. These include intoxications, metabolic and endocrine disorders, head trauma, and cerebral bleeding. It is important to note here that encephalitis, as any other organic condition, may occur in patients who have preexisting psychiatric disorders. Differential diagnosis in such instances may become difficult.

MANAGEMENT AND TREATMENT

Management of intracranial infections often requires hospitalization and treatment with specific antimicrobial agents. Isolation may be required in certain infections. Supportive measures with fluids and pain killers are provided as needed. When psychiatric symptoms arise, psychotropic agents may be used. In cases of delirium and psychosis, high-potency antipsychotic agents can be used with caution to alleviate psychiatric symptoms and control behavior. Antidepressant medications may be used as deemed appropriate. Sedative and benzodiazepines should be avoided since they may increase the clouding of the consciousness.

Chronic sequelae such as dementia or personality changes may not be responsive to pharmacological treatment. Ritalin may be given to some patients with postencephalitic syndrome who present with lethargy, mental slowing, and drowsiness. Anticonvulsant agents may be needed to control epilepsy or other impulsive behavior. Antiparkinsonian agents may be needed to treat postencephalitic parkinsonism. Behavioral management and rehabilitation can be beneficial in some cases. In all instances, supportive psychotherapy can be helpful.

13

PSYCHIATRIC MANIFESTATIONS OF ENDOCRINE DISORDERS

The relationship between emotional symptoms and hormonal changes has long been recognized and documented by clinicians and researchers. Endocrine disorders such as thyroid and adrenal diseases are capable of causing a wide variety of psychiatric symptoms. Physiological hormonal changes such as those occurring prior to menstruation, during pregnancy, and during menopause are also known to produce several psychiatric and behavioral manifestations which may vary among women depending on several other factors.

Although the exact mechanism by which hormonal abnormalities produce changes in mental functions and personality is still not fully understood, it is well known that hormonal systems are closely linked to neurotransmitter systems. Therefore, hormonal changes are likely to influence the release of serotonin, norepinephrine, dopamine, and several other neurotransmitters, leading to various psychiatric symptoms. Conversely, psychiatric disorders are likely to influence the release of various hormones such as cortisol, growth hormones, prolactin, and others that may complicate the clinical picture.

HYPERTHYROIDISM

Hyperthyroidism refers to a syndrome resulting from excessive production of thyroid hormones. The condition can be caused by several diseases, such as thyroid tumors, inflammation, and spontaneous diffuse overactivity of the gland. Severe stress, and acute emotional disturbances have been implicated in precipitating hyperthyroidism as well (Michael & Gibbons, 1963). Common physical signs and symptoms include fatigue, palpitations, tremor, diarrhea, weight loss despite increased appetite, excessive sweating, intolerance of warm temperatures, and oligomenorrhea (reduced menstrual blood flow). In cases of Graves' disease, prominent proptosis (exophthalmos or protrusion of the eyes) may occur. The gland may or may not be enlarged. The disease affects females more than males in a ratio of 6 to 1, and occurs most commonly during the second and third decades of life (Lishman, 1987).

Psychiatric manifestations of hyperthyroidism include restlessness, irritability, overactivity, and emotional lability. Distractibility, impaired concentration, and difficulty with recent memory may occur as well (Whybrow, Prange & Treadway, 1969). In some cases, severe anxiety and panic symptoms can develop. The symptoms can be identical to those encountered in "primary" disorders to the point that misdiagnosis is fairly common. Symptoms of mood disorders can also occur, especially mania and, less frequently, depression. Symptoms of psychosis with hallucinations and delusions that can resemble schizophrenia have also been reported (Greer & Parsons, 1968).

Careful differential diagnosis should be undertaken, and the diagnosis is usually confirmed by specific laboratory tests that show elevation of thyroid hormones. Treatment should focus on the underlying cause by administering antithyroid drugs. Usually, most neuropsychiatric symptoms reverse with antithyroid treatment, although a full year may be needed before complete recovery is attained (Goldman,1992). Symptomatic treatment with anxiolytic and antipsychotic agents may be required, and is often very effective.

HYPOTHYROIDISM

Hypothyroidism or myxedema refers to a syndrome resulting from decreased production of thyroid hormones. The condition can be caused by autoimmune disorders, ablation of the gland as a result of surgery or radioactive treatment, and, in some cases, long-term lithium therapy. Common signs and symptoms include sluggishness, low energy level, vague generalized aches, muscle weakness, slow pulse, weight gain despite diminished appetite, intolerance to cold temperatures, constipation, menorrhagia (increased menstrual blood flow) in females, and impotence in males. The skin becomes dry with a pale puffy complexion. The eyelids are baggy due to the edema which involves the face and limbs. Hair loss often occurs, and its texture is usually lank and dry. Speech is slow and the voice is coarse and toneless. The gland may or may not be enlarged. Reflexes are often diminished. The disease occurs more frequently in females than in males in a ratio of 8 to 1, and is more common during middle age (Lishman, 1987).

Psychiatric symptoms are fairly common and may precede all other physical signs and symptoms. Typical manifestations are those of mental lethargy and slowing of all cognitive functions, leading to poor concentration and impairment of short-term memory. There is profound loss of interest and initiative, with a tendency towards apathy. In severe or long-standing cases, marked dementia develops and patients report losing things and making "stupid" mistakes (Goldman, 1992). Depressive symptoms and, to some extent, anxiety may commence as early as three weeks after the onset of hypothyroidism (Denicoff et al., 1990). Insomnia, irritability, and mood lability often occur. Psychosis is usually nonspecific and often involves hallucinations and delusions. The symptoms can occur either in the context of an acute delirium or as a progressive subacute psychotic syndrome that may resemble schizophrenic disorders. Undetected hypothyroidism in infancy can lead to profound mental retardation. Therefore, thyroid tests are conducted routinely nowadays at birth to prevent such devastating complications.

Hypothyroidism should be differentiated from "primary" depression and psychoses and from different types of dementia. The diagnosis can be confirmed by laboratory tests that reveal low thyroid hormones. Treatment consists of replacement with thyroid hormones, depending on blood levels. Almost complete recovery of cognitive and affective deficits can be expected with thyroid replacement in patients with severe hypothyroidism within six months of therapy. Such deficits in patients with moderate or mild hypothyroidism are less likely to respond to thyroid replacement. Psychotropic agents such as antipsychotic and antidepressant medications may be warranted in certain cases. Antipsychotic agents have been reported to be effective in controlling psychotic symptoms. However, many believe that affective symptoms are resistant to treatment with antidepressant medications (Goldman, 1992).

CUSHING'S SYNDROME

Cushing's syndrome refers to a disease resulting from excessive production of cortisol, a hormone produced by the adrenal gland. The disease can be primary, arising from tumors of the adrenal gland itself, or secondary, resulting from increased secretion of ACTH by the pituitary gland. ACTH stimulates the adrenal gland, causing bilateral hyperplasia of the gland, which leads to the excessive production of cortisol. Secondary type comprises about 80% of all cases. In addition, the syndrome can be caused by chronic administration of corticosteroids in the course of treatment or due to abuse by some athletes and others. Symptoms include fatigue, muscle weakness, oligomenorrhea (decreased menstrual blood flow) in females and impotence in males, hirsutism (increased hair growth), moon facies, hypertension, and hyperglycemia (elevated blood sugar). Typically, patients gain weight, mostly around the trunk. The skin may become pigmented and excessive bruising is common.

The disease is more common in women than in men, and starts usually in the third or fourth decade of life (Goldman, 1992). Many cases have been noted to start during pregnancy, at puberty, or at menopause. It has also been reported to occur in people who are subjected to prolonged periods of psychological stress (Lishman, 1987).

Depression and anxiety are seen in about half the patients with Cushing's syndrome. Common symptoms include sense of sadness, insomnia, poor concentration, somatic preoccupation, and suicidal tendencies. Hypomanic and manic symptoms are less common in Cushing's syndrome, yet they occur often in cases of excessive oral intake of steroids. Psychosis occurs in about 20% of cases. Paranoid delusions as well as auditory and visual hallucinations with or without delirium have been reported. Cognitive changes are also common, yet they may not be as pronounced as affective symptoms (Goldman,1992).

The disease should be differentiated from other mood disorders and psychoses. Other conditions that cause cognitive impairment should be entertained. The diagnosis can be confirmed by laboratory investigations showing high cortisol levels. Treatment is usually surgical to remove the tumor or part of the enlarged gland. Cushing's syndrome resulting from treatment with corticosteroids can be reversed by gradual withdrawal of the drug, although relapse of certain symptoms may occur due to the withdrawal itself. Psychiatric symptoms tend to improve significantly following proper treatment. Psychotropic medications such as antipsychotic agents and lithium can be effective in controlling psychosis and mania. However, tricyclic antidepressants may exacerbate depression secondary to hypercortisolism. In such instances, electroconvulsive therapy (ECT) may prove beneficial (Reus,1987).

ADDISON'S DISEASE

Addison's disease or adrenal insufficiency refers to the syndrome resulting from decreased production of cortisol. The disease can be caused by failure of the pituitary gland to produce ACTH or by atrophy of the adrenal gland itself due to autoimmune disease or acute adrenal failure. Symptoms include fatigue, weakness, anorexia, vomiting, and weight loss. Other features include, low blood pressure, skin pigmentations and amenorrhea (absence of menstruation) in women, and impotence in men. The disease occurs more frequently in males than in females and appears to strike people in early adult to middle life.

Psychiatric manifestations include depressive symptoms with emotional withdrawal, apathy, and loss of initiative. Anxiety, irritability, and suspiciousness can also occur. Symptoms resembling anorexia nervosa have been reported. Occasionally, progressive dementia can develop. In certain instances, frank delirium with visual hallucinations, paranoia, and bizarre posturing can occur (Jefferson & Marshal, 1981).

The disease needs to be differentiated from "primary" psychiatric disorders and mental disorders due to other medical conditions that present with similar features. Major depression and anorexia nervosa, in particular, should be ruled out. The diagnosis can be confirmed by laboratory tests that shows low cortisol levels. Treatment consists of replacement therapy with adequate dosages of steroids, which usually leads to quick reversal of most physical and psychiatric symptoms. The use of psychotropic agents for symptomatic relief may be beneficial as well.

PHEOCHROMOCYTOMA

Pheochromocytoma is a tumor of the adrenal medulla that leads to excessive secretion of norepinephrine and epinephrine, leading to a severe sympathetic response. Symptoms include palpitation, lightheadedness, flushing, sweating, dizziness, tremulousness, tightness in the chest, nausea and vomiting, headache, and elevation in blood pressure. Severe anxiety with panic are very common, and may resemble generalized anxiety disorder and panic disorder to a large extent. The patient becomes fearful and overwhelmed with feeling of impending death. The symptoms usually occur in the form of sudden attacks lasting from a few minutes to several hours. The disease should be differentiated from panic disorder and generalized anxiety disorder. Hyperthyroidism may at times present with similar symptoms. The diagnosis can be made by identifying increased levels of catecholamines or their metabolites in the blood or urine. Treatment is usually by surgical removal of the tumor.

HYPERPARATHYROIDISM

Hyperparathyroidism refers to excessive production of parathyroid hormone, often caused by benign tumors involving parathyroid glands. The main disturbance of this disorder involves high calcium blood levels. This, in turn, produces a series of signs and symptoms. Patients usually suffer from kidney stones, bone fractures and muscular weakness, and wasting. Other symptoms include anorexia, nausea, constipation, headache, increased thirst, and polyuria (frequent urination). Women are affected more often than men, especially those of middle age.

Psychiatric manifestations occur in about two-thirds of patients (Petersen, 1968). Symptoms include depression and lack of energy, with occasional outbursts of tension and irritability. Suicidality is not uncommon, and several completed suicides have occurred. Other patients present with dementia, including poor memory, general mental slowing, and personality changes. Occasionally, acute delirium with disorientation, hallucinations, paranoia, and agitation can occur (Goldman, 1992).

The disorder should be differentiated from "primary" mood disorders and other disorders that cause delirium or dementia. The diagnosis can be confirmed by laboratory tests that reveal elevation of calcium and parathyroid hormone blood levels. Treatment is usually by surgical removal of the tumors. Most physical and psychiatric symptoms resolve fairly quickly. Antidepressant medications may be useful in certain cases of severe depression.

HYPOPARATHYROIDISM

Hypoparathyroidism refers to reduced production of parathyroid hormone. The most common cause is removal of the glands accidentally during thyroid and other neck surgeries. Other causes include autoimmune disease involving the parathyroid glands and familial absence or degeneration of the glands. It can also occur in association with Addison's disease. Typically, serum calcium level is low, creating symptoms of fatigue, tetany (muscle spasm), facial grimacing, and numbness and tingling in the hands and feet or around the mouth. Typical and atypical seizures are frequent. Cataract may occur at an early age.

Psychiatric symptoms occur in at least half the patients (Denko & Kaelbling, 1962). The most frequent disturbances involve acute "organic" reactions with features typical of delirium. Other psychiatric symptoms include anxiety, panic attacks, depression, and mood changes. Occasionally, symptoms of presenile dementia develop.

The disorder should be differentiated from anxiety, panic, and mood disorders. Dementia, hysteria, and epilepsy should also be considered in the differential diagnosis. Treatment with calcium supplements is often very successful. Seizures are treated with anticonvulsant agents if needed. Psychotropic medications may be used depending on the clinical presentation.

DIABETES MELLITUS

Diabetes mellitus results from an absolute or relative deficiency of insulin production by the pancreas, causing disturbance in carbohydrate metabolism and elevation of blood glucose level and glycosuria (sugar in the urine). This leads to a series of clinical symptoms, including fatigue, excessive thirst, and polyuria (excessive urination). Patients become more susceptible to infections. Complications of diabetes mellitus include neuropathy (degeneration of peripheral nerves), retinopathy (damage to the retina with potential blindness), and nephropathy (kidney damage). Atherosclerotic vascular changes are common. Very high glucose blood level can lead to diabetic ketoacidosis and diabetic coma. High doses of insulin or failure to consume adequate amount of calories can result in hypoglycemia and coma as well. The disease can strike in childhood or later in life. Genetic factors and obesity predispose to the illness. Severe emotional stress can aggravate the disorder, and may sometimes bring the disorder into being (Lishman, 1987).

Psychiatric symptoms can occur as a result of vascular changes within the brain. Symptoms of depression, psychosis, and dementia have been reported. Delirium can occur in cases of diabetic ketoacidosis or hypoglycemia. Symptoms may include agitation, disorientation, paranoia, and visual hallucinations. In addition, a hypoglycemic attack may mimic to a large extent a panic attack.

Patients with diabetes tend to become angry and depressed, and react with various psychological defenses in an attempt to deal with their illness. Patients go through phases of rebellion with wilful neglect of treatment. This is particularly common among diabetic adolescents who often refuse to adhere to their diet or don't administer their insulin as instructed. Diabetes in children can disrupt parent-child relationships and create a series of reactions, including guilt, anxiety, resentment, and dependency. In adults, issues of marriage and sexual performance are of prime importance. Decreased sexual interest, impotence in men, and amenorrhea (absence of menstruation) in women are common.

The disease can be diagnosed by laboratory blood tests showing consistently high glucose levels. Various psychiatric disorders such as depression and anxiety disorders can occur independently in diabetic patients, and should be treated vigorously since emotional stress—like physical stress—can exacerbate diabetes and raise insulin requirement. The disease can be managed by dietary restrictions, weight loss, and the use of oral hypoglycemic agents or insulin. Patient and family education is essential. Psychotherapy and support groups can be helpful. The use of psychotropic medications may be indicated depending on the severity of the psychiatric symptoms.

PREMENSTRUAL SYNDROME

Premenstrual syndrome or PMS has received serious attention in the past few years due to its high prevalence and the significant impact it may have on the functioning of millions of women. DSM-IV (1994) has included this condition under the name Premenstrual Dysphoric Disorder as a proposed category needing further study and research. This diagnosis does not apply to mild cases that have minimal effect on the woman's social or occupational functioning. The condition presumably results from hormonal changes that occur during the latter part of the luteal phase of the menstrual cycle. The disorder has also been reported in nonmenstruating women who have had a hysterectomy but retain ovarian function. The age of onset may be at any time after menarche. However, most patients seeking treatment are usually over the age of 30.

Most women report mood changes with irritability, dysphoria, anxiety, and outbursts of anger. In some cases, insomnia and other symptoms of severe depression occur. Most symptoms resolve a few days after the onset of menses, only to appear again before the next period. When the symptoms don't resolve within a few days of the onset of menses, the possibility of another psychiatric diagnosis should be entertained. Physical symptoms that accompany PMS include breast tenderness, headaches, joint or muscle pain, and a sensation of "bloating."

The disorder can be diagnosed based on the history and the pattern of occurrence in women during the menstrual cycle. It should be differentiated from other psychiatric disorders such as major depression or anxiety disorders. These disorders tend to last longer and do not follow the specific cyclic pattern of PMS. Most cases do not require psychotropic medications, but the use of the new antidepressants (Prozac, Zoloft, and Paxil) and anxiolytics has proven effective in many cases. Psychotherapy can be useful in certain patients.

14

PSYCHIATRIC MANIFESTATIONS OF METABOLIC AND VITAMIN DEFICIENCY DISORDERS

Any serious interference with the normal metabolic process of the brain can lead to several neurological and psychiatric changes. The symptoms often occur in the course of encephalopathy, which refers to acute generalized involvement of the brain with certain pathological processes. Examples include hepatic encephalopathy and renal encephalopathy. In other instances, psychiatric symptoms develop following chronic metabolic changes that affect brain tissue over a long period of time. Examples include chronic cerebral hypoxia and vitamin deficiency diseases. Metabolic disorders are likely to interfere with various neurotransmitter systems, leading to corresponding behavioral and mental changes

LIVER DISEASE

Hepatic failure can be acute or chronic. Acute causes include severe infection of the hepatitis B or non A non B types, exposure to hepatotoxic drugs or anesthetic agents, and acute hepatic vein occlusion (Scharschmidt, 1985). Chronic causes include liver cirrhosis secondary to alcoholism or malnutrition, Wilson's disease, and cancer of the liver. Hepatic encephalopathy often presents with symptoms of delirium (see Chapter Two). The condition can progress to stupor, then coma. Patients show characteristic flapping tremor involving the wrists and fingers (asterixis). Focal neurological signs and abnormal reflexes can be observed.

Psychiatric symptoms are mostly those encountered during delirium and they include irritability, increased psychomotor activity, visual and auditory hallucinations, and paranoid delusions. In chronic hepatic failure, psychiatric symptoms may commence insidiously and may mimic schizophrenia, anxiety, and mood disorders. Cognitive impairment and personality changes can also develop in certain long-standing cases.

Hepatic encephalopathy should be differentiated from mental disorders due to other medical conditions, "primary" psychoses, mood disorders, and dementias. The diagnosis can be confirmed by laboratory tests showing high ammonium blood levels. EEG recordings show generalized slowing of brain waves. The appearance of characteristic triphasic waves signals poor prognosis. Treatment consists of restriction of protein intake and the administration of oral antibiotics to decrease the formation of bacterial ammonia in the gut. Most symptoms can be reversible if early treatment is implemented. The prognosis can vary and often depends on the degree of liver damage. Psychotropic medications, especially sedatives, should be avoided since they may exacerbate hepatic encephalopathy. In cases when a tranquilizer must be used, lorazepam (Ativan) may be given in small doses (Kraus et al., 1987).

RENAL FAILURE

Like hepatic failure, renal failure can be acute or chronic. Common causes of renal failure include autoimmune disease, infection, severe dehydration or shock following burns or crush injuries, and exposure to toxic agents. Other causes include diabetes mellitus, systemic lupus erythematosus, and chronic lithium therapy. Renal failure leads to elevation of urea level in the blood, causing what is known as uremia. Symptoms include fatigue and lethargy, nausea and vomiting, and peripheral neuropathy. High urea levels can cause uremic encephalopathy, which is virtually similar to hepatic encephalopathy with symptoms of delirium (see Chapter Two). Stupor followed by coma can develop in untreated cases. Epileptic fits occur in about one third of cases.

Psychiatric symptoms encountered in delirium include irritability, agitation, disorientation, hallucinations, and delusions. In addition, psychiatric symptoms can precede the development of encephalopathy and occur during periods of clear sensorium. These include lethargy, anorexia, depression, and, occasionally, psychosis. Mental sluggishness and impaired cognitive functions may mimic early dementia. It is worth noting here that patients with chronic kidney failure who require hemodialysis usually suffer from chronic depression and often become angry and hostile because of their disability. In addition, some of these patients may develop what is known as dialysis dementia, which may be caused by high concentration of aluminum in the brain. Furthermore, some patients who undergo hemodialysis may suffer from a different kind of delirium with psychosis due to cerebral edema caused by the dialysis itself, especially if the dialysis is performed rapidly (Levy, 1981; Jack, Robin & McKinney, 1983/1984).

The diagnosis can be made by laboratory tests showing high blood level of urea along with other signs of renal failure. EEG recordings resemble those seen in hepatic encephalopathy, and epileptic disturbances may appear. Renal encephalopathy should be differentiated from other encephalopathies and toxic conditions. Treatment requires hemodialysis along with supportive medical management. Depression, whether due to uremia or to patients' reaction to their illness, should be identified and treated.

Individual psychotherapy and support groups can be very helpful. Psychotropic medications may be used with caution, and frequent blood level monitoring is essential. Lithium therapy should be discontinued in cases of lithium-induced kidney disease.

ELECTROLYTE DISTURBANCES

Any disruption in the balance of water and electrolytes can lead to significant physiological abnormalities that can cause a series of physical and mental changes. Disorders that can cause electrolyte imbalance include water intoxication, water depletion, renal failure, endocrine disorders, pulmonary diseases, and diabetes mellitus. Physical symptoms depend on the underlying etiologic factor and they are beyond the scope of this book. Delirium occurs frequently, and may be followed by stupor and coma in some cases.

Psychiatric symptoms may develop during the course of delirium or they may occur insidiously during states of clear sensorium. Symptoms of anxiety, depression, psychosis, and cognitive deficits have been reported (Lishman, 1987).

The disorder is diagnosed by blood tests that show abnormal levels of sodium, potassium, calcium, magnesium, zinc, or carbon dioxide. Other medical causes of mental disorders should be ruled out. "Primary" psychiatric disorders such as anxiety, depression, or psychosis need to be differentiated from the condition. Treatment consists of correcting the underlying electrolyte imbalance.

HYPOGLYCEMIA

Hypoglycemia refers to the state of low blood sugar. Physiological hypoglycemia occurs during fasting periods. In certain individuals, hypoglycemic attacks can be precipitated in response to the ingestion of large amounts of carbohydrate, which induces excessive secretion of insulin. Such conditions are considered benign and present with mild physical and mental changes. Pathological hypoglycemia, on the other hand, can bring serious consequences. Causes include insulin-secreting pancreatic tumors (insulinoma), liver disease, endocrine diseases, and overdose on insulin or oral hypoglycemic agents. Insulin overdose can occur accidentally in diabetic patients. Some healthy individuals may abuse such agents for the purpose of getting attention or experiencing a certain type of pleasure. Symptoms of insulinoma include intermittent attacks of dizziness, lightheadedness, restlessness, feelings of hunger, sweating, and palpitation. Brief episodes of unconsciousness may occur and epileptic attacks can be provoked. In severe cases, coma may follow (Lishman, 1987).

Psychiatric symptoms of hypoglycemia are mostly those of anxiety and panic attacks. Depersonalization, derealization, disorientation, and odd behavior occur frequently. Occasionally, psychotic symptoms with paranoid delusions may develop. Amnesia for the events occurring during the attack may occur, raising the suspicion of hysterical reactions. In chronic cases, memory along with other cognitive functions may become impaired, leading to dementia and personality changes (Marks, 1981).

The diagnosis is made by measuring blood sugar levels. EEG abnormalities may be found. "Primary" anxiety and panic disorders should be ruled out. Other conditions that need to be considered in the differential diagnosis include hysteria, dementia, epilepsy, and mental disorders due to other medical conditions. Treatment is accomplished by restoring normal glucose blood level, either through the administration of sugar or by adjusting insulin dosage. Pancreatic tumors may require surgical intervention.

CEREBRAL ANOXIA

Cerebral anoxia or hypoxia refers to the state of decreased oxygenation of the brain. Causes include chronic obstructive pulmonary diseases (COPD) such as emphysema and chronic bronchitis, heart disease, cerebral vascular disease, severe anemia, exposure to high altitudes, and carbon monoxide poisoning.

Symptoms of acute cerebral anoxia include confusion, disorientation, and, in severe cases, impairment of consciousness. Delirium with psychomotor agitation, severe anxiety, hallucinations, and delusions has been reported. Memory loss is a common occurrence after transient episodes of acute cerebral anoxia. Brain damage with various neurological sequelae or death may occur if cerebral anoxia continues more than three to five minutes, as in cases of asphyxiation or drowning. Chronic cerebral anoxia often causes mild mental disorder with symptoms of inattentiveness, decreased concentration, slowing of thought process, impaired motor coordination, and subtle alterations in judgment. Irritability, anxiety, or depression may also be present. Long-term complications include cognitive impairment, dementia, and personality changes. Complete recovery can be expected if proper oxygenation of the brain is restored before brain damage commences. Treatment should be directed at the underlying cause; however, oxygen therapy may be needed.

ACUTE PORPHYRIA

Acute intermittent porphyria is a genetic metabolic disease that affects the metabolism of porphyrins. The illness is inherited as a dominant autosomal gene with limited penetrance and declares itself mostly in the third decade of life. The episodes are precipitated by the ingestion of alcohol and certain drugs, especially barbiturates. Symptoms include attacks of severe abdominal pain, nausea, vomiting, headache, and severe constipation. Epileptic fits, weakness, and numbness in the limbs develop rapidly.

Psychiatric symptoms occur in 25%–75% of cases and can dominate the clinical picture. They include emotional lability, depression, restlessness, and violent behavior. Clouding of consciousness or delirium with hallucinations and delusions can occur. In some cases, ongoing psychotic symptoms resembling schizophrenia have been reported. The diagnosis is confirmed by the detection of excess porphobilinogen in the urine. No specific treatment is available. Patients should avoid alcohol and drugs that precipitate the attack. Psychotic symptoms may be treated effectively with trifluoperazine (Lishman, 1987).

PELLAGRA

Pellagra results from subacute nicotinic acid deficiency. The syndrome involves gastrointestinal symptoms, skin lesions, and psychiatric disturbances. Patients complain of anorexia, insomnia, nervousness, dizziness, headache, palpitations, and paraesthesiae. Depressive symptoms of severe nature can occur with considerable risk of suicide. Cognitive impairment with poor memory and confabulation develop at later stages. Occasionally, prolonged severe nicotinic acid deficiency leads to florid psychotic manifestation with violent outbursts, hallucinations, and paranoid delusions. Dramatic recovery usually occurs in response to treatment with nicotinic acid (Lishman, 1987).

VITAMIN B12 DEFICIENCY

Vitamin B12 deficiency leads to pernicious anemia, degeneration of the spinal cord, and psychiatric syndromes. A wide variety of psychiatric disorders have been reported in connection with vitamin B12 deficiency. These include depression, psychosis, delirium, and dementia (Zucker et al., 1981). It is believed that symptoms occur due to either associated anemia that may affect brain functions or physiological and structural changes that take place in the absence of vitamin B12. Diagnosis is confirmed by laboratory test that shows low blood level of vitamin B12. "Primary" psychiatric disorders and mental disorders due to other medical conditions need to be considered in the differential diagnosis. Treatment with vitamin B12 injections often brings dramatic relief

FOLIC ACID DEFICIENCY

Folic acid deficiency leads to megaloblastic anemia, which may be associated with polyneuropathies, fatigue, depression, and progressive dementia. The diagnosis can be confirmed by laboratory test showing low blood level of folic acid. Mental disorders due to other medical conditions should be differentiated from folic acid deficiency syndrome. Treatment is usually successful by the use of folic acid. Often, vitamin B12 may need to be given as well since both vitamins seem to be involved in the metabolic disturbances. Compared to other depressed patients, folate deficient depressives were found to respond less favorably to antidepressant medications or electroconvulsive therapy (Reynolds et al., 1970).

WERNICKE'S ENCEPHALOPATHY AND KORSAKOFF'S PSYCHOSIS

These syndromes are associated with thiamine deficiency and alcoholism. They are discussed in Chapter Sixteen.

15

PSYCHIATRIC MANIFESTATIONS OF EXPOSURE TO TOXIC SUBSTANCES AND PHARMACOLOGICAL AGENTS

Acute or chronic exposure of the central nervous system to poisonous agents or drugs may result in a wide variety of psychological, behavioral, and cognitive changes. The clinical picture is often similar to other mental disorders caused by medical conditions, although, in some instances, it may mimic a "primary" psychiatric disorder. In addition, physical and neurological signs and symptoms often occur, depending on the nature of the underlying poisonous agent. The psychoactive effects of these substances probably result from a complicated interaction that takes place between the toxic substance and various neurotransmitter systems.

I. METAL POISONING

Lead Poisoning

Lead can be present in water, food, air, dust and soil in small quantities that normally do not pose any significant health hazard. However, lead poisoning can occur when the person is exposed to high levels of lead and the intake of lead exceeds the ability of the body to eliminate it. Lead can contaminate drinking water while passing through lead pipes and can also contaminate food kept for a long time in lead-containing pots. Most common cases of lead poisoning occur in children due to the ingestion of lead-based paint used on toys and furniture and from old houses. Occupational intoxication occurs mostly via inhalation of lead by workers dealing with materials containing lead used by various industries.

Children are usually susceptible to acute lead poisoning, which may commence in the form of encephalopathy. In such instances, symptoms of delirium with visual and auditory hallucinations often occur. Convulsions and coma may follow in severe cases. Chronic subclinical exposure of children has been found to cause reduction in IQ scores, with academic and cognitive deficits (Needleman et al., 1990). Symptoms of chronic exposure are more common in adults and they include fatigue, arthralgia, abdominal pain, anorexia, and constipation. Peripheral neuropathy and paralysis of various muscles can occur in some cases. Psychiatric manifestations include depression, euphoria, nervousness, irritability, hallucinations, and delusions (Cullen, Robins & Eskenazi, 1983).

The diagnosis is usually confirmed by positive history of being exposed to lead and by laboratory tests that show high lead blood levels. Disorders that can mimic lead encephalopathy include hepatic and uremic encephalopathies and encephalitis. Treatment is accomplished by the administration of a chelating agent such as BAL or EDTA to help eliminate lead from the body.

Symptoms may be relieved with treatment, and most changes may be reversed if treatment is undertaken early in the process. However, in cases of severe lead encephalopathy in children, especially when treatment is delayed, brain damage may occur, leaving the child with blindness, epilepsy, cerebral palsy, or mental retardation (Perlstein & Attala, 1966).

Arsenic Poisoning

Arsenic is a tasteless, odorless metal that can be found naturally in the environment and is used in several industries. Acute arsenic poisoning commonly occurs following accidental, suicidal, or homicidal ingestion, while chronic poisoning often results from occupational exposure.

Symptoms of acute poisoning include having a metallic taste and garlic breath odor, vomiting, diarrhea, and abdominal cramps. Delirium, seizures, coma, and death may follow within days. Symptoms of chronic poisoning include skin lesions, anorexia, weight loss, headache, vertigo, apathy, and mental confusion. Peripheral neuropathy with pain, paraesthesia, and motor weakness occurs in most cases. Psychiatric symptoms include anxiety, depression, psychosis, and personality changes. Severe memory impairment can develop and may mimic Korsakoff's psychosis (Gross & Nagy, 1992).

The diagnosis can be made based on the detection of high levels of arsenic in the blood and urine. Treatment consists of gastric lavage and giving activated charcoal. Chelating agents such as BAL and penicillamine can be helpful. Supportive medical measures may be essential in some cases. Early detection and treatment may minimize possible neurological sequelae.

Mercury Poisoning

Acute or chronic mercury poisoning can still occur in several industrial settings, mainly due to inhalation of toxic fumes or absorption through contaminated skin. In the past, most cases of toxicity occurred among felt hat workers, giving rise to the expression "mad as a hatter." At present, some industries still utilize mercury preparations, leading to occasional cases of mercury poisoning. High-risk groups include miners, smelters, jewelers, photographers, dentists, and makers of mirrors, instruments, and batteries.

Physical symptoms include headache, insomnia, fatigue, stomatitis, gingivitis, excessive salivation, coarse tremor, neuropathy, and other neurological deficits. Psychiatric symptoms include irritability, mood lability, depression, hallucinations, decreased sexual drive, impaired cognition and judgment, withdrawal, and excessive shyness.

Mercury poisoning should be suspected when some of the symptoms described above emerge in persons with history of exposure to mercury. The diagnosis is confirmed by blood and urine tests showing high mercury levels. Treatment consists of supportive medical measures and the administration of chelating agents such as BAL or penicillamine. Improvement can be expected, but in severe cases central and peripheral nervous system damage may be irreversible (Gross & Nagy, 1992).

Manganese Poisoning

Manganese poisoning is strictly an occupational disease that occurs mostly among miners and workers who process manganese ores. Exposure to manganese can also occur in several industries involved in the manufacturing of steel, dry batteries, paints, ceramic, glass, ink, dyes, matches, welding rods, fungicides, and fertilizers. Manganese poisoning is relatively rare despite common exposure. It is believed that a large quantity of manganese must be absorbed before harmful effects are produced (Lishman, 1987).

Physical symptoms include headache, anorexia, fatigue, increased sleep, and impotence. Psychiatric symptoms may precede all other manifestations and can occur in up to 70% of cases. They include uncontrollable laughters and crying, aberrant behavior, forgetfulness, mental dullness, depression, irritability, emotional lability, and outbursts of rage. Occasionally, hallucinations and delusions occur. Parkinsonian symptoms consisting of tremor, rigidity, mask-like facies, slow movements, and gait disturbances also occur.

The diagnosis can be made based on history of exposure and on detecting high manganese levels in the blood and urine. Treatment is accomplished by removing the individual from the toxic environment, although symptoms may persist for several weeks after. Using a chelating agent such as EDTA may accelerate recovery. The use of L-dopa may be useful in alleviating parkinsonian symptoms. Recovery can be expected in some cases, but permanent brain damage can occur in severe cases.

II. ORGANOPHOSPHATES

Organophosphates are used as insecticides and for chemical warfare in what is known as "nerve gas." They act as anticholinesterases leading to accumulation of acetylcholine in the central nervous system, which results in neurotoxicity. Exposure is often accidental, but suicidal and homicidal cases have been reported. The poison can enter the body through skin contamination, inhalation, or ingestion.

The onset of action is within minutes or hours from the time of exposure. Symptoms include headache, giddiness, drowsiness, tremor, slurred speech, ataxia, and generalized weakness. Severe toxicity can lead to coma and eventually to death. Psychiatric manifestations include restlessness, anxiety, mood lability, depression, apathy, confusion, increased dreaming, memory and concentration deficits, and psychosis.

The diagnosis can be made based on positive history of exposure and laboratory tests showing inhibition of cholinesterase in red blood cells. Treatment is accomplished by giving adequate dosage of atropine, removing contaminated clothing, and washing exposed skin surfaces. With prompt and successful treatment, full recovery is expected. However, some survivors may continue to experience symptoms of irritability, depression, poor memory, and psychosis for extended periods of time (Ellenhorn & Barceloux, 1988).

III. CARBON MONOXIDE POISONING

Carbon monoxide is a colorless and odorless gas that is often undetectable and is formed from incomplete combustion of organic matter. It is considered to be the leading cause of poisoning death in the United States, accounting for about 4000 deaths a year (Ellenhorn & Barceloux, 1988). Common sources include car exhaust fumes, inadequately ventilated furnaces, defective heating equipment and cigarette smoking. Poisoning is often accidental, although suicidal poisoning is fairly common.

Carbon monoxide binds firmly to hemoglobin, displacing oxygen and causing serious brain anoxia. Early symptoms include headache, dizziness, fatigue, irritability, and dimming of vision. As the level of carbon monoxide rises in the blood, delirium with disorientation and alteration in the level of consciousness develop. Later, unconsciousness, coma, and convulsions occur, and death soon follows.

If the patient recovers from acute poisoning within less than an hour of the intoxication, the chances of permanent neurological or psychiatric sequelae are very small. In some cases, initial apparent full recovery may be followed by sudden relapse of neurological and psychiatric symptoms within two to four weeks (Myers, Snyder & Emhoff, 1985). In cases where patients survive severe or prolonged carbon monoxide poisoning, permanent brain damage may occur. Common neurological sequelae include parkinsonism and seizure disorder. Common psychiatric sequelae include memory impairment, depression, apathy, and personality changes. Most of the neuropsychiatric sequelae, except memory deficits and gait disturbances, often recover after one year.

The diagnosis is made based on history of exposure and clinical features that often correlate with carbon monoxide levels in the blood. Treatment is accomplished by removing the person from the source of the poisoning into fresh air. Oxygen therapy should be initiated as soon as possible. Supportive medical measures are provided as needed. Younger patients have higher chances of complete recovery following carbon monoxide hypoxic unconsciousness. Loss of consciousness is not always necessary for developing delayed neurological or psychiatric sequelae (Gross & Nagy, 1992).

IV. MEDICATIONS: SIDE EFFECTS AND TOXICITY

Most medications prescribed in clinical practice are capable of adversely affecting the central nervous system and producing significant changes in the patient's mood, perception, thinking, cognition, behavior, and sleep pattern. The effects of such agents vary considerably from one patient to another and depend on the dose, the age of the patient, the underlying physical and psychological conditions, and several other biological and environmental factors. Psychiatric side effects of pharmacological agents include delirium, depression, mania, hallucinations, delusions, cognitive impairment, and behavioral disturbances. It is believed that such agents produce psychiatric abnormalities through their interference with various neurotransmitter systems.

Antidepressant Medications

It is widely known that prescribing antidepressant medications for some depressed patients with manic depressive disorder can precipitate a manic episode. Furthermore, antidepressant medications have been reported to activate psychotic symptoms in schizophrenic patients. They have also been implicated in causing psychotic symptoms, including hallucinations and paranoid delusions in depressed patients who had no prior history of psychosis or mania. Antidepressants that have been reported to cause such side effects include imipramine, amitriptyline, doxepin, amoxapine, maprotiline, trazodone, bupropion, and MAO inhibitors (Asaad, 1990). New antidepressants (Prozac, Zoloft, Paxil) are capable of producing psychotic or manic responses as well.

Benzodiazepines

These agents are used for anxiety and panic disorders. They are also used as hypnotics for sleep disturbances. Benzodiazepines, like alcohol, have a depressant effect on the central nervous system. They can cause depressive symptoms, excitement, agitation, nightmares, and disorientation. Older patients are particularly at a high risk of developing mental confusion and cognitive impairment. Furthermore, several benzodiazepines have been implicated in causing short-term memory disturbances. Occasionally, benzodiazepines have been found to cause hallucinations and paranoid delusions.

Withdrawal from benzodiazepines resembles to a great extent alcohol withdrawal, and may present with delirium, and visual and auditory hallucinations, and can lead to seizures (Asaad, 1990). Benzodiazepine abuse and withdrawal are discussed further in Chapter Seventeen.

Lithium

Lithium is used for bipolar disorders, depression, and impulse control disorders. At therapeutic blood levels, lithium can cause mild depressive feeling. In addition, visual hallucinations have been reported in response to lithium treatment (Sandyk & Gillman, 1985). When lithium levels are within toxic range, symptoms and signs of delirium may develop. These include alteration in the level of consciousness, agitation, disorientation, sedation, slurred speech, nausea, vomiting, and tremor. Stupor and coma may follow. Patients with preexisting schizophrenia or brain damage seem to be more prone to developing such side effects during lithium therapy (Paulseth & Klawans, 1985).

Central Stimulants

Stimulants include amphetamines, methylphenidate (Ritalin), and pemoline (Cylert). These agents are used for the treatment of attention deficit disorder, narcolepsy, appetite suppression, and, sometimes, depression. Central stimulants produce sympathomimetic effects, with increased pulse rate, elevated blood pressure, diaphoresis, dilated pupils, and tremor. Psychiatric symptoms include increased excitability, euphoria, irritability, anxiety, and insomnia. At higher doses, or in cases of prolonged use, paranoid delusions, thought disorder, and hallucinations have been reported (Paulseth & Klawans, 1985).

Anticonvulsants

Anticonvulsants are used for different types of epilepsy, bipolar disorders, and impulse control disorders. They include phenytoin (Dilantin), carbamazepine (Tegretol), ethosuximide (Zarontin), and valproic acid (Depakote). Visual, auditory, and tactile hallucinations and delusions have been reported as side effects to anticonvulsant medications (Asaad, 1990). At toxic levels, these medications can cause delirious states, ataxia, and nystagmus.

Antiparkinsonian Agents

Drugs that are used in the treatment of Parkinson's disease increase the concentration of dopamine in the central nervous system and, consequently, produce florid psychotic symptoms or delirium. Examples of these drugs include levodopa, carbidopa, amantadine, and bromocriptine. Hallucinations, especially of the visual modality, paranoid delusions, disorientation, and confusion have been reported in many patients. Mood changes with severe depression and hypomania also occur in certain patients. Antipsychotic agents that block dopamine receptors may alleviate the psychosis, yet often exacerbate the symptoms of Parkinson's disease. The new antipsychotic clozapine has been found to be fairly effective in controlling psychotic symptoms without worsening the parkinsonian syndrome (Friedman & Lannon, 1989).

Anticholinergic Agents

Many drugs, including antidepressants and antipsychotic agents, possess high anticholinergic properties. Benztropine (Cogentin) and trihexyphidyl (Artane), commonly used in conjunction with antipsychotic agents to counteract extrapyramidal side effects, are frequent causes of anticholinergic toxicity. Clinical presentation consists of rapid pulse, elevated temperature, dry skin and mucous membranes, urinary retention, constipation, blurred vision, and dilated pupils. Psychiatric symptoms consist of delirium with visual and tactile hallucinations, paranoia, disorientation, and agitation. Lilliputian hallucinations where people or objects are seen greatly reduced in size may be present. The elderly seem to be more vulnerable to anticholinergic toxicity, even at lower doses (Paulseth & Klawans, 1985). Treatment may be accomplished by repeated injections of a cholinergic agent such as physostigmine.

Antihistamines and Decongestants

Most antihistamines and over-the-counter drugs that are used for cold, cough, or insomnia are capable of causing depression, mental slowing, and disorientation. Visual hallucinations have been reported in association with such agents (Asaad, 1990). At toxic doses, delirium may occur. It is important to note here that many antihistamines possess strong anticholinergic properties which may contribute to the toxic effects, as well.

Analgesics and Antiinflammatory Agents

Morphine and other opiate derivatives are capable of causing hallucinatory symptoms. Aspirin and phenacetin may produce toxicity at high doses which may manifest with disorientation, agitation, and hallucinations (Cummings & Miller, 1987). Indocin is known to cause toxic reactions, with headache, agitation, ataxia, depression, and hallucinations (Mills, 1974). Corticosteroids can cause mood changes ranging from hypomania to severe depression. Psychosis has also been reported as a side effect to steroidal therapy.

Cardiovascular Agents

Several drugs that are used for heart diseases and hypertension have been shown to produce a wide range of psychiatric and behavioral disturbances, especially in the older population. Symptoms can occur in the course of a full-blown delirium or as isolated symptoms in states of clear consciousness. Visual hallucinations have been reported as side effects to digoxin, propranolol, timolol, clonidine, isosorbide dinitrate, quinidine, reserpine, and methyldopa (Asaad, 1990). In addition, depression has been reported in association with several agents, including propranolol, procainamide, hydralazine, reserpine, and methyldopa.

Miscellaneous Drugs

Several other drugs have been reported to cause various psychotic symptoms, especially visual hallucinations. These include cimetidine, ranitidine, disulfiram, ketamine, nitrous oxide, hormones, antineoplastic agents, and antimicrobial agents (Asaad, 1990).

16

ALCOHOL-INDUCED MENTAL DISORDERS

Several psychiatric symptoms have been described in association with syndromes resulting from prolonged alcohol consumption and repeated withdrawal episodes. These symptoms include hallucinations, delusions, depression, delirium, behavioral disturbances, cognitive impairment, and personality changes. Physical and neurological signs and symptoms often occur as well.

BIOLOGICAL CONSIDERATIONS

Alcohol has a depressant effect on the central nervous system similar to that of benzodiazepines, barbiturates, and anesthetic agents. Initially, alcohol exerts its effect on the reticular formation, leading to increased excitability and mild euphoria. Later, it acts on the cortical neurons, causing sedation and depressive symptoms. It is likely that alcohol intoxication and withdrawal disrupt the equilibrium among various neurotransmitter systems, leading to mood changes, psychotic phenomena, and behavioral disturbances.

Withdrawal from alcohol can lead to series of episodes, including delirium tremens, hallucinations, and seizures. The exact mechanism of delirium tremens and hallucinatory phenomena in association with alcoholism is not known. Ballenger and Post (1978) suggested that repeated heavy alcohol intake over prolonged periods of time may create "kindling" effects on the brain. They elaborated that this will lead to long-term changes in the neuronal excitability and, consequently, produce the symptoms of alcohol withdrawal and delirium tremens. More recently, Hemmingsen et al. (1988) indicated that regional cerebral blood flow is increased and seems to correlate significantly with the onset of visual hallucinations and agitation in patients during alcohol withdrawal.

Nutritional deficiencies that may be associated with chronic alcohol abuse are likely to produce serious brain abnormalities such as Wernicke's encephalopathy, Korsakoff's psychosis, and dementia. Thiamine deficiency seems to play a central role in these conditions.

ALCOHOL INTOXICATION

Alcohol may induce different symptoms in different individuals, depending on the level of tolerance and biological vulnerability. Alcohol intoxication refers to a mental disorder characterized by behavioral changes with disinhibition of sexual or aggressive impulses, irritability, mood changes, and impaired judgment. Physical symptoms include slurred speech, unsteady gait, and muscle incoordination. Amnesia of the events occurring during the period of intoxication (blackout) may occur in certain cases. Alcohol blood level may determine the degree of intoxication. Death can occur in cases of severe intoxication due to suppression of respiration or aspiration of vomitus. Alcohol intoxication may mimic intoxication due to sedatives and hypnotic agents. Treatment is achieved by detoxification using benzodiazepines and thiamine for several days.

PATHOLOGICAL INTOXICATION

This condition is also known as alcohol idiosyncratic intoxication. The essential feature of this condition is that the patient may react to a relatively small amount of alcohol with severe violence or unpredictable behavior. The behavior is often atypical of the person when not drinking, and is followed by amnesia of the event. It is believed that certain underlying brain dysfunction may predispose to this condition. This disorder has been omitted from DSM-IV because of lack of supportive evidence that the disorder is distinct from alcohol intoxication.

ALCOHOL WITHDRAWAL

Alcohol withdrawal occurs in individuals who drink heavily for prolonged periods of time and who stop drinking or reduce the amount they usually consume. The symptoms usually start several hours after cessation of or reduction in alcohol intake. Uncomplicated alcohol withdrawal is characterized by coarse tremor of hands and face, anxiety, irritability, headache, and insomnia. Tachycardia, elevation of blood pressure and sweating are common signs. In some instances, grand mal seizures may occur. Withdrawal from benzodiazepines or barbiturates tend to resemble alcohol withdrawal syndrome. Complicated alcohol withdrawal may commence in the form of delirium tremens or alcohol hallucinosis.

I. Delirium Tremens

This condition is currently referred to in DSM-IV(1994) as Alcohol Withdrawal Delirium. The syndrome usually begins on the second or third day after the cessation of or reduction in drinking. However, in some cases, the symptoms may begin as early as one day or as late as one week after abstinence. These symptoms include clouding of consciousness, disorientation, tremulousness, irritability, hallucinations, agitation, and elevation of blood pressure.

The onset is usually sudden, and often at night. Early signs of perceptual disturbances include hyperexcitability, startle responses, and vivid nightmares. Transient illusions and hallucinations follow, accompanied by intense anxiety. Illusions become more pronounced. Spots on the wall may be mistaken for spiders, and cracks in the ceiling may be perceived as snakes. Vivid visual hallucinations of people or small animals are particularly common. Tactile hallucinations are also common. Typically, patients report feeling small animals or insects crawling over their skin. This condition is known as "formication." Tactile hallucinations of similar nature occur frequently in cases of cocaine and amphetamine intoxication (Asaad, 1990). Auditory hallucinations occur less frequently in alcohol withdrawal delirium, and usually consist of threatening or persecutory voices. Unlike alcohol hallucinosis, these auditory hallucinations occur in states of clouded consciousness as part of delirium.

Delirium tremens should be recognized and treated promptly as a medical emergency due to the significant mortality rate associated with the condition. Patients must be admitted to the hospital and should be placed on appropriate level of observation to prevent possible injuries to self or others. Fluid and electrolyte abnormalities should be corrected. Vitamins, especially thiamine, should be administered as soon as possible. Proper detoxification regimen with benzodiazepines needs to be implemented promptly. Agitation, anxiety, and hallucinatory symptoms usually respond well to benzodiazepines, but antipsychotic medications may be needed in some cases (see Chapter Two).

II. Alcohol Hallucinosis

The term "hallucinosis" generally refers to hallucinations that occur in a clear state of consciousness and that are caused by physical factors. This disorder is classified in DSM-IV under "Alcohol-Induced Psychotic Disorders." Alcohol hallucinosis presents mainly with auditory hallucinations that persist after the person has recovered from the acute symptoms of alcohol withdrawal and is no longer drinking. The symptoms usually appear within the first 48 hours of abstinence, but sometimes they may be delayed for one or two weeks. Typically, the first onset follows 10 years or more of heavy drinking. Hallucinations may begin as simple unformed noises such as buzzing, mumbling, or cracking sounds, and later progress into more complex and elaborate auditory hallucinations. The voices may address the patient directly, but more often they discuss him or her in the third person. In some instances, they may command the patient to harm self or others. Patients appear to be in clear distress and react to their hallucinations with fear and apprehension. Visual hallucinations have also been reported as part of alcohol hallucinosis syndrome.

In most cases, the hallucinations last for only a few hours, and disappear completely in a few days. However, in about 10% of the patients, the hallucinations can last for weeks or months, and may become chronic in rare cases. In some patients, other psychotic symptoms such as ideas of reference and poorly systematized persecutory delusions develop. Furthermore, illogical thinking with tangential associations and inappropriate affect can occur at a later stage, making the clinical presentation virtually indistinguishable from schizophrenia.

Alcohol hallucinosis usually responds well to antipsychotic medications. However, in some patients, the hallucinations may persist or show little response to treatment. Tegretol or lithium may be effective in some cases. Occasionally, ECT may be needed in those cases that persist beyond a few weeks (Asaad, 1990).

WERNICKE'S ENCEPHALOPATHY

Wernicke's encephalopathy represents an acute neuropsychiatric reaction to severe thiamine deficiency, which may result from chronic alcohol consumption and poor dietary intake. The syndrome starts abruptly, presenting mainly with mental confusion, ataxia and ophthalmoplegia (eye movement abnormalities). In some patients, perceptual distortions and various types of hallucinations develop. Such hallucinations are usually transient and are much milder than those observed in delirium tremens. Occasionally, Wernicke's encephalopathy develops simultaneously with delirium tremens (Lishman, 1987).

Wernicke's encephalopathy is treated with large doses of thiamine, in addition to other measures taken in the treatment of delirium tremens as outlined above. Untreated cases can lead to mortalities or turn into Korsakoff's psychosis. Reuler, Girard & Cooney (1985) reported that approximately 80% of patients with Wernicke's encephalopathy who survive develop Korsakoff's psychosis.

KORSAKOFF'S PSYCHOSIS

Korsakoff's psychosis or syndrome represents the chronic untreated form of Wernicke's encephalopathy. It is characterized by memory disturbances and confabulation. Significant personality deterioration and social impairment may follow. The term "psychosis" associated with this entity is probably misleading since no formal psychotic symptoms such as hallucinations or delusions are reported as part of the syndrome. In fact, DSM-IV (1994) classifies Korsakoff's syndrome under "Alcohol-Induced Persisting Amnestic Disorder" (see Chapter Three). No effective treatment is available for Korsakoff's syndrome, however, Martin et al. (1989) reported that fluvoxamine, a serotonin reuptake inhibitor, may offer some promise in reducing memory deficits in some patients.

ALCOHOL DEMENTIA

In some instances, prolonged and heavy ingestion of alcohol may lead to global deterioration in cognitive abilities and a clinical presentation similar to that seen in dementia. This condition may be difficult to distinguish from other types of dementias (see Chapter Three).

DIFFERENTIAL DIAGNOSIS

Alcohol abuse is often associated with other underlying psychiatric disorders such as mood disorders, anxiety and panic disorders, and certain personality disorders. Patients who suffer from both a substance abuse disorder and a psychiatric condition are often labeled as having a "dual diagnosis." It is essential to identify such conditions since specific treatment must be implemented to correct the underlying disturbances. In some instances, specific measures can also prevent the relapse of alcohol abuse, especially in those patients who self-medicate with alcohol to alleviate their symptoms of anxiety, depression, or paranoia.

Hallucinations that occur in the course of delirium tremens or alcohol hallucinosis need to be differentiated from other types of hallucinations that may be caused by "primary" psychiatric disorders such as schizophrenia or mania. Surawicz (1980) offered a few guidelines to help differentiate alcohol hallucinosis from schizophrenia. He suggested that the onset of alcohol hallucinosis occurs later in life, commonly between age 40 and 60, and the first episode occurs typically after 10 years or more of heavy drinking. Unlike schizophrenia, alcohol hallucinosis often appears suddenly towards the end of an extended period of alcohol intoxication, as alcohol blood level begins to drop. In addition, patients with alcohol hallucinosis usually do not exhibit a thought disorder or delusional thinking. Although in some instances alcohol hallucinosis can become chronic and persist for years, most cases, unlike schizophrenia, resolve within weeks or months.

17

DRUG-INDUCED MENTAL DISORDERS

Drugs have been known and used by man for medical and recreational purposes throughout recorded history. The recent explosion in drug use, including cocaine, heroin, and hallucinogens, has presented society and the medical community with a difficult challenge. In the past decade, a large body of evidence has accumulated in support of short-term and long-term damaging effects of such agents on the brain.

Psychoactive substances seem to exert profound affects on the central nervous system and produce a variety of behavioral, emotional, and cognitive changes in certain individuals. Consequently, various psychiatric syndromes have been reported in association with the use of recreational drugs. These include mood disorders, anxiety and panic disorders, paranoid states, and hallucinations. Furthermore, intoxication and withdrawal reactions may precipitate a series of physical signs and symptoms, as well. The exact mechanism by which drugs produce various psychiatric symptoms is still not fully understood. Current thinking points toward major alterations and imbalances among various neurotransmitter systems, including serotonin, norepinephrine, dopamine, acetylcholine, endorphins, and others.

HALLUCINOGENS

Hallucinogens or psychedelic (mind-realizing) drugs refer to a group of chemical substances that are capable of producing perceptual distortions and a wide variety of other psychiatric symptoms. These drugs include LSD, mescaline, psilocybin, DMT, MDA, DOM, and others. Syndromes induced by hallucinogens include hallucinosis, delusional disorder, mood disorder, and "flashbacks."

Under the influence of LSD, perceptions become brilliant and intense. All of the senses are enhanced and the individual is usually more attentive to details. Colors and textures seem richer. Visual distortions and illusions are common. Soon, visual hallucinations of simple or complex nature develop. Auditory and tactile hallucinations are experienced on rare occasions. Synesthesia, where various forms of hallucinations are experienced simultaneously, are particularly common. Changes in body image and alterations in the perception of time and space, including depersonalization and derealization, also occur. Physical symptoms include pupillary dilation, tachycardia, sweating, palpitations, blurring of vision, tremor, and incoordination. Hallucinations usually begin within one hour of the drug ingestion and last for six hours to three days. Severe anxiety, panic, and psychosis may be present, creating what is known as a "bad trip." Severe intoxication with hallucinogen can lead to delirious states in some individuals (Asaad, 1990).

Delusional states can be induced by hallucinogenic drugs. This condition often accompanies or follows the hallucinosis syndrome. The course is usually brief; however, long episodes of delusional states resembling schizophrenic disorders have been reported. Depressive symptoms occur shortly after hallucinogen use. Usually they begin within one to two weeks and persist for more than 24 hours after cessation of such use. Depressive symptoms may resemble "primary" depression and may be difficult to distinguish from preexisting depressive symptoms.

Hallucinogen Persisting Perception Disorder, or "flash-backs," refers to spontaneous recurrences of visual hallucinations and illusions that occur in individuals who have a history of repeated ingestion of drugs. These experiences occur during a drug-free period and resemble those hallucinations experienced during the active stage of drug use. Flashbacks occur in about 25% of all psychedelic drug users and may commence several months after the last use of the drug. They are most likely to occur under stress, or with fatigue, alcohol intoxication, or severe illness. The intensity and frequency of flashbacks tend to decrease with time in most cases (Asaad, 1990).

PHENCYCLIDINE (PCP)

Phencyclidine, or PCP, is a white crystal that can be manufactured easily and is known on the street as "angel dust" or "crystal." PCP may be taken by mouth, smoked, snorted, or injected intravenously. On the market, there are about 30 different preparations related to PCP. Ketamine, a short-acting anesthetic, is a related drug with psychoactive properties similar to those of PCP. These drugs are capable of producing a wide variety of psychiatric syndromes, including delirium, delusional disorder, hallucinosis, and mood disorders.

PCP intoxication presents initially with elevated blood pressure, nystagmus, diminished responsiveness to pain, ataxia, dysarthria, and diaphoresis. Psychiatric symptoms include euphoria, bodily warmth, tingling, peaceful floating sensations, and depersonalization. Later, striking alterations in body image, distortions of space and time perception, and synesthesia occur. Auditory and visual hallucinations, as well as paranoid delusions, develop in some instances. Severe anxiety, agitation, assaultiveness, or bizarre behavior may be observed in some individuals.

Symptoms usually last for few hours to one day; however, some patients may remain psychotic for as long as two weeks (Asaad, 1990). In severe cases of intoxication,

delirium may develop (see Chapter Two). In some instances, delusional disorder of paranoid nature, depression, or anxiety may be seen in reaction to using PCP in the
absence of acute signs or symptoms of intoxication. These
disorders need to be differentiated from "primary" disorders for the purpose of providing appropriate treatment.

INHALANTS AND VOLATILE SOLVENTS

The abuse of inhalants and volatile solvents has spread
excessively in recent years, especially among adolescents.
This category of drugs includes varnish removers, gaso-
line, lighter fluid, glues, rubber cement, cleaning fluids,
aerosols such as spray paint, and others. The active
ingredients that appear to be responsible for the addictive
behavior include toluene, benzene, and halogenated hy-
drocarbons. These agents cause euphoria, excitement, a
floating sensation, and a sense of heightened power. Some
patients experience hallucinations, mood lability, and
personality changes. Other symptoms include dizziness,
slurred speech, ataxia, belligerence, assaultiveness, and
impaired judgment.

The onset of symptoms is usually within a few minutes
after the inhalation, and the experience lasts for an hour or
two. In cases of severe intoxication, convulsions and coma
can develop and death may occur due to central nervous
system depression or cardiac arrhythmia. Prolonged heavy
use can lead to irreversible brain damage (Ellenhorn &
Barceloux, 1988).

OPIOIDS

The term opioids is now used to refer to a large number
of chemically diverse narcotic substances that seem to
bind specifically to opioid receptors and produce specific
actions. Examples include heroin, morphine, demerol,
methadone, buprenorphine, pentazocine, butorphanol,

and nalbuphine. Intoxication with opioids causes initial euphoria followed by apathy and dysphoria. Physical findings include pupillary constriction, drowsiness, slurred speech, and impaired attention and memory. Hallucinations have also been reported in cases of opioids toxicity (Asaad, 1990). Withdrawal from opioids causes nausea and vomiting, lacrimation or runny nose, pupillary dilation, yawning, sweating, piloerection, fever, and insomnia (DSM-IV, 1994).

COCAINE

Cocaine acts on the central nervous system almost instantly. Initially, the user experiences euphoria and a sense of well being. Later, grandiosity, hypervigilance, agitation, and impaired judgment occur. Physical symptoms include tachycardia, pupillary dilation, elevated blood pressure, perspiration or chills, and nausea and vomiting. In cases of severe intoxication, confusion, rambling, anxiety, and apprehension are likely to be present. Occasionally, some patients may develop a psychotic disorder and experience persecutory delusions that may last for a week or longer.

Hallucinations have also been reported in the course of cocaine intoxication. Most frequently, patients report tactile hallucinations consisting of insects crawling up the skin (formication). Visual hallucinations may also occur and often consist of seeing small animals or insects. Auditory hallucinations are reported less frequently in association with cocaine intoxication (Siegel, 1978).

After the immediate effects of cocaine have subsided, patients experience unpleasant rebound effects which make up what is known as the "crash." Symptoms include dysphoria, anxiety, irritability, tremulousness, fatigue, hypersomnia, depression, and craving for cocaine. If the symptoms extend beyond 24 hours, the condition is referred to as cocaine withdrawal.

Severe cocaine intoxication may lead to delirium, which may develop within 24 hours of intake of cocaine. Cocaine is now believed to be highly addictive, and the administration of large doses may result in syncope, chest pain, and seizures. Death may occur due to cardiac arrhythmias or respiratory paralysis.

MARIJUANA

Marijuana is also known as cannabis, hashish, pot, kif, and bhang. The active ingredient of the plant is known as tetrahydrocannabinol (THC). Intoxication occurs almost immediately after one smokes the substance, peaks within half an hour, and usually lasts about three hours. Symptoms consist of euphoria, sensation of slowed time, anxiety, paranoia, impaired judgment, and social withdrawal. Occasionally, patients experience panic attacks, dysphoric moods and inappropriate laughters. Some patients report feelings of "dying" or "losing their minds" In cases of severe intoxication, distortions of time, space, and body parts may occur. Depersonalization, derealization, increased sensitivity to sound, synesthesia, and true hallucinations may be experienced. In rare instances, some patients develop a psychotic disorder consisting of persecutory delusions that commence shortly after the use of marijuana and may last for a few days. Physical symptoms include tachycardia, increased appetite, dry mouth, and conjunctival injection. Long-term heavy users of marijuana may develop tolerance and may experience mild withdrawal symptoms upon abstaining from smoking the plant. However, there is no clinical evidence that the drug causes any significant addictive problems among chronic users (Millman, 1989).

AMPHETAMINES AND OTHER STIMULANTS

Amphetamines and similar stimulants such as methylphenidate (Ritalin) and pemoline (Cylert) can cause

a series of physical, psychological, and behavioral disturbances. Symptoms of intoxication include irritability,
anxiety, dysphoria, agitation, and insomnia. Some patients experience paranoid delusions and visual, tactile,
and auditory hallucinations. Physical findings include
tachycardia, elevated blood pressure, pupillary dilation,
perspiration or chills, and nausea and vomiting. Amphetamine intoxication resembles to a great extent cocaine
intoxication. Severe intoxication can lead to delirium (see
Chapter Two). Withdrawal symptoms also resemble cocaine withdrawal and consist of dysphoric mood, anxiety,
depression, fatigue, and insomnia or hypersomnia.

BARBITURATES AND BENZODIAZEPINES

Sedatives, hypnotics and anxiolytics have a depressant
effect on the central nervous system similar to that of
alcohol. Therefore, symptoms of intoxication or withdrawal associated with these drugs can be very similar to
alcohol intoxication or withdrawal respectively, including withdrawal delirium (see Chapter Sixteen). Hallucinations, delusions, and amnestic disorder have been
reported in association with sedatives, hypnotics, and
anxiolytic intoxication or withdrawal. Furthermore, grand
mal seizures can occur in cases of withdrawal from large
doses of these agents.

TREATMENT CONSIDERATIONS

Intoxications and withdrawals from various drugs are
best managed by the implementation of specific detoxification regimens that are appropriate, depending on the
type of drug and clinical presentation. Hallucinations and
delusions may respond favorably to benzodiazepines.
However, the use of small doses of high potency
antipsychotic agents, such as haloperidol, may be needed
and is usually highly effective in certain cases. Depressive
symptoms also respond very well to antidepressant medi-

cations. Drug rehabilitation and NA meetings may be needed in patients with a history of chronic drug abuse or dependence.

REFERENCES

Addonizio, G. (1989). The patient with Parkinson's Disease. In *Treatment of Psychiatric Disorders (Vol. 2)*. Washington, DC: American Psychiatric Association.

Alexopoulos, G. S. (1989). The patient with epilepsy. In *Treatment of Psychiatric Disorders (Vol. 2)*. Washington, DC: American Psychiatric Association.

Asaad, G. (1990). *Hallucinations in Clinical Psychiatry: A Guide for Mental Health Professionals*. New York: Brunner/Mazel.

Ballenger, J. C. & Post, R. M. (1978). Kindling as a model for alcoholic withdrawal syndrome. *British Journal of Psychiatry,* 133, 1–14.

Barraclough, B. (1981). Suicide and epilepsy. In E. H. Reynolds and M. R. Trimble (Eds.), *Epilepsy and Psychiatry*. Edinburgh: Churchill Livingstone.

Crow, T. J. (1978). Viral causes of psychiatric disease. *Postgraduate Medical Journal,* 54, 763–767.

Cullen, M. R., Robins, J. M., & Eskenazi, B. (1983). Adult inorganic lead intoxication: Presentation of 31 new cases and a review of recent advances in the literature. *Medicine,* 62, 221–247.

Cummings, J. L. (1985). *Clinical Neuropsychiatry*. Orlando, FL: Grune & Stratton.

Cummings, J. L. (1992). Neuropsychiatric aspects of Alzheimer's disease and other dementing illnesses. In S. C. Yudofsky & R. E. Hales (Eds.), *Textbook of Neuropsychiatry (Second Edition)*. Washington, DC: American Psychiatric Press.

Cummings, J. L. & Miller, B. L. (1987). Visual hallucinations—clinical occurrence and use in differential diagnosis. *Western Journal of Medicine,* 146, 46–51.

Denicoff, K. D., Joffe, R. T., Lakshmanan, M. C., et al. (1990). Neuropsychiatric manifestations of altered thyroid state. *American Journal of Psychiatry*, 147, 94–99.

Denko, J. D. & Kaelbling, R. (1962). The psychiatric aspects of hypoparathyroidism. *Acta Psychiatrica Scandinavica*, supplement, 164, 1–70.

Department of Health and Human Services (1989). *Interagency Head Injury Task Force Report*. Washington, DC: Government Printing Office.

Diagnostic and Statistical Manual of Mental Disorders, Fourth Edition (1994). Washington, DC: American Psychiatric Association.

Ellenhorn, M. J. & Barceloux, D. G. (1988). *Medical Toxicology: Diagnosis and Treatment of Human Poisoning*. New York: Elsevier Science.

Fallon, B. A., Nields, J. A., Parsons, B., et al. (1993). Psychiatric manifestations of Lyme borreliosis. *Journal of Clinical Psychiatry*, 54, 7, 263–268.

Flor-Henry, P. (1969). Psychosis and temporal lobe epilepsy: A controlled investigation. *Epilepsia*, 10, 363–395.

Folstein, S. E.(1989). *Huntington's Disease: A Disorder of Families*. Baltimore, MD: Johns Hopkins University Press.

Folstein, M. F., Folstein S. E., & McHugh, P. R. (1975). Mini-mental state. A practical method for grading the cognitive state of patients for the clinician. *Journal of Psychiatric Research*, 12, 189–198.

Friedman, J. H. & Lannon, M. C. (1989). Clozapine in the treatment of psychosis in Parkinson's Disease. *Neurology*, 39, (9), 1219–1221.

Gastaut, H. & Broughton, R. (1972). *Epileptic Seizures: Clinical and Electrographic Features, Diagnosis and Treatment*. Springfield IL: Charles C. Thomas.

Goldman, M. B. (1992). Neuropsychiatric features of endocrine disorders. In S. C. Yudofsky & R. E. Hales

(Eds.), *Textbook of Neuropsychiatry (Second Edition)*. Washington DC: American Psychiatric Press.

Greer, S. & Parsons, V. (1968). Schizophrenia-like psychosis in thyroid crisis. *British Journal of Psychiatry,* 114, 1357–1362.

Gross, L. S. & Nagy, R. M. (1992). Neuropsychiatric aspects of poisonous and toxic disorders. In S. C. Yudofsky & R. E. Hales (Eds.), *Textbook of Neuropsychiatry (Second Edition)*. Washington, DC: American Psychiatric Press.

Gusella, J., Wexler, N. S., Conneally, P. M., et al. (1983). A polymorphic DNA marker genetically linked to Huntington's disease. *Nature,* 306, 234–239.

Hemmingsen, R., Vorstrup, S., Clemmesen, L., et al. (1988). Cerebral blood flow during delirium tremens and related clinical states studied with Xenon-133 inhalation tomography. *American Journal of Psychiatry,* 145, 11, 1384–1390.

Jack, R., Rabin, P. L., & McKinney, T. D. (1983/1984). Dialysis encephalopathy: a review. *International Journal of Psychiatry and Medicine,* 13, 309–326.

Jarvik, L. F. (1981). Hydergine as a treatment for organic brain syndrome in late life. *Psychopharmacology Bulletin,* 17, 40–41.

Jefferson, J. J. & Marshal, J. R. (1981). *Endocrine Disorders, in Neuropsychiatric Features of Medical Disorders*. New York: Plenum.

Kaplan, R. F., Meadows, M. E., Vincent, L. C., et al. (1992). Memory impairment and depression in patients with Lyme encephalopathy. *Neurology,* 42, 7, 1263–1267.

Katon, W. & Raskind, M. (1980). Treatment of depression in the medically ill elderly with methylphenidate. *American Journal of Psychiatry,* 137, 963–965.

Kraus, J. M., Desmond, P. V., Marshall J. P., et al. (1987). Effects of aging and liver disease on disposition of lorazepam. *Clinical Pharmacology and Therapy,* 24, 411–419.

Kreutzer, J. S. & Zasler, N. D. (1989). Psychosexual consequences of traumatic brain injury: methodology and preliminary findings. *Brain Injury,* 3, 177–186.

Levy, N. B. (1981). Psychological reactions to machine dependency: hemodialysis. *Psychiatric Clinics of North America,* 4, 351–363.

Lipowski, Z. J. (1980-a). Organic Mental Disorders: introduction and review of syndromes. In H. I. Kaplan, A. M. Freedman, & B. J. Sadock (Eds.), *Comprehensive Textbook of Psychiatry, Third Edition.* Baltimore: Williams and Wilkins.

Lipowski, Z. J. (1980-b). *Delirium: Acute Brain Failure in Man.* Springfield, IL: Charles C. Thomas.

Lishman, W. A. (1987). *Organic Psychiatry: The Psychological Consequences of Cerebral Disorder (Second Edition).* Oxford: Blackwell Scientific Publications.

Liston, E. H. (1984). Diagnosis and management of delirium in the elderly patient. *Psychiatric Annals,* 14, 109–118.

Markowitz, J. C. & Perry, S. W. (1992). Effects of Human Immunodeficiency Virus on the central nervous system. In S. C. Yudofsky & R. E. Hales (Eds.), *Textbook of Neuropsychiatry (Second Edition).* Washington, DC: American Psychiatric Press.

Marks, V. (1981). Symptomatology. In V. Marks & F. C. Rose, *Hypoglycaemia (Second Edition).* Oxford: Blackwell Scientific Publications.

Marotta, R. & Perry, S. (1989). Early neuropsychological dysfunction caused by the human immunodeficiency virus. *Journal of Neuropsychiatry and Clinical Neurosciences,* 1, 225–235.

Martin, P. R., Adinoff, B., Eckardt, M. J., et al. (1989). Effective pharmacotherapy of alcoholic amnestic disorder with fluvoxamine. *Archive of General Psychiatry,* 46, 617–621.

Masters, C. L., Harris, J. O., Gajdusek, D. C., et al. (1979). Creutzfeldt-Jakob disease: patterns of worldwide occurrence and the significance of familial and sporadic clustering. *Annals of Neurology,* 5, 177–188.

McKinlay, W. W., Brooks, D. N., Bond, M. R., et al. (1981). The short-term outcome of severe blunt head injury as reported by relatives of the injured person. *Journal of Neurology, Neurosurgery and Psychiatry,* 44, 527–533.

Meyers, B. S. & Young, R.C. (1989). Dementia of the Alzheimer type. In *Treatment of Psychiatric Disorders (Vol. 2).* Washington DC: American Psychiatric Association.

Michael, R. P. & Gibbons, J. L. (1963). Interrelationships between the endocrine system and neuropsychiatry. *International Review of Neurobiology,* Vol. 5, 243–302.

Millman, R. (1989). Cannabis abuse and dependence. In *Treatment of Psychiatric Disorders (Vol. 2).* Washington DC: American Psychiatric Association.

Mills, J. A. (1974). Non-steroidal antiinflammatory drugs. Part II. *New England Journal of Medicine,* 290, 1002–1005.

Misra, P. C. & Hay, G. G. (1971). Encephalitis presenting as acute schizophrenia. *British Medical Journal,* 1, 532–533.

Mjones, H. (1949). Paralysis agitans: a clinical and genetic study. *Acta Psychiatrica Scandinavica,* 54, 1–195.

Mora, G. (1980). Historical and theoretical trends in psychiatry. In H. I. Kaplan, A. M. Freedman, & B. J. Sadock (Eds.), *Comprehensive Textbook of Psychiatry, Third Edition.* Baltimore: Williams and Wilkins.

Myers, R. A. M., Snyder, S. K., & Emhoff, T. A. (1985). Subacute sequelae of carbon monoxide poisoning. *Annals of Emergency Medicine,* 14, 1163–1167.

Navia, B. A., Jordan, B. D., & Price, R. W. (1986). The AIDS dementia complex, I: Clinical features. *Annals of Neurology,* 19, 517–524.

Needleman, H. L., Schell, A., Bellinger, D., et al. (1990). The long-term effects of exposure to low doses of lead in childhood: an 11 year follow-up report. *New England Journal of Medicine,* 322, 83–88.

Neppe, V. M. & Tucker, G. J. (1992). Neuropsychiatric
    aspects of seizure disorders. In S. C. Yudofsky & R. E.
    Hales (Eds.), *Textbook of Neuropsychiatry (Second
    Edition).*Washington, DC: American Psychiatric Press.
Paulseth, J. E. & Klawans, H. L. (1985). Drug-induced
    behavioral disorders. In P. J. Vinken, G. W. Bruyn, &
    H. L. Klawans (Eds.), *Handbook of Clinical Neurol-
    ogy, Vol. 2. Neurobehavioral Disorders.* Amsterdam:
    Elsevier.
Peele, T. L. (Ed.) (1977). *The Neuroanatomical Basis for
    Clinical Neurology.* New York: McGraw-Hill.
Perlstein, M. & Attala, R. (1966). Neurologic sequelae of
    plumbism in children.*Clinical Pediatrics,*5, 292–298.
Petersen, P. (1968). Psychiatric disorders in primary
    hyperparathyroidism. *Journal of Clinical Endocri-
    nology and Metabolism,* 28, 1491–1495.
Plotkin, D. A. & Jarvik, L. F. (1986). Cholinergic dysfunc-
    tion in Alzheimer's disease: Cause or effect? In J. M.
    Van Ree & S. Matthysse (Eds.), *Perspectives in
    Aetiology of Psychiatric Disorders: Brain Neurotrans-
    mission and Neuropeptides, Vol. 65.* Amsterdam:
    Elsevier.
Pond, D. A. & Bidwell, B. H. (1960). A survey of epilepsy
    in 14 general practices, II: Social and psychological
    aspects. *Epilepsia,* 1, 285–299.
Price, R. W., Brew, B., Sidtis, J., et al. (1988). The brain in
    AIDS: central nervous system HIV-1 infection and
    AIDS dementia complex. *Science,* 239, 586–591.
Price, T. R. P., Goetz, K. L., & Lovell, M. R. (1992).
    Neuropsychiatric aspects of brain tumors. In S. C.
    Yudofsky & R. E. Hales (Eds.), *Textbook of
    Neuropsychiatry (Second Edition).* Washington, DC:
    American Psychiatric Press.
Reuler, J. B., Girard, D. E., & Cooney, T. G. (1985). Wernicke's
    encephalopathy. *New England Journal of Medicine,*
    312, 1035–1039.
Reus, V. I. (1987). Disorders of the adrenal cortex and
    gonads. In C. B. Nemeroff & P. T. Loosen (Eds.),

Handbook of Clinical Psychoneuroendocrinology. New York: Guilford.

Reynolds, E. H., Preece, J. M., Bailey, J., & Coppen, A. (1970). Folate deficiency in depressive illness. *British Journal of Psychiatry, 117*, 287–292.

Robinson, R. G., Starr, L. B., Kubos, K. L., et al. (1983). A two-year longitudinal study of poststroke mood disorders: Findings during the initial evaluation. *Stroke, 14*, 736–741.

Robinson, R. G., Kubos, K. L., Starr, L. B., et al. (1984). Mood disorder in stroke patients: Importance of lesion location. *Brain, 107*, 81–93.

Robinson, R. G., Bolduc, P. L., & Price, T. R. (1987). Two-year longitudinal study of poststroke mood disorders: Diagnosis and outcome at one and two years. *Stroke, 18*, 837–843.

Roelcke, U., Barnett, W., Wilder-Smith, E., et al. (1992). Untreated neuroborreliosis: Bannwarth's syndrome evolving into acute schizophrenia-like psychosis. A case report. *Journal of Neurology, 239*, 3, 129–131.

Ruff, R. M., Marshall, L. F., Klauber, M. R., et al. (1990). Alcohol abuse and neurological outcome of the severely head injured. *Journal of Head Trauma Rehabilitation, 5*, 21–31.

Sandyk, R. & Gillman, M. A. (1985). Lithium-induced visual hallucinations: Evidence for possible opioid mediation. *Annals of Neurology, 17* (6), 619–620.

Scharschmidt, B. F. (1985). Acute and chronic hepatic failure with encephalopathy. In J. B. Wyngaarden & L. H. Smith (Eds.), *Cecil's Textbook of Medicine, 17th Ed.* Philadelphia: W. B. Saunders.

Siegel, R. K. (1978). Cocaine hallucinations. *American Journal of Psychiatry, 135*, 309–314.

Silver, J. M., Hales, R. E., & Yudofsky, S. C. (1992). Neuropsychiatric aspects of traumatic brain injury. In S. C. Yudofsky & R. E. Hales (Eds.), *Textbook of Neuropsychiatry (Second Edition).* Washington, DC: American Psychiatric Press.

Singer, S. F. & Read, S. L. (1989). The patient with stroke. In *Treatment of Psychiatric Disorders, (Vol. 2).* Washington, DC: American Psychiatric Association.

Spar, J. E. (1989). Organic personality syndrome. In *Treatment of Psychiatric Disorders, (Vol. 2).* Washington, DC: American Psychiatric Association.

Starkstein, S. E. & Robinson, R. G. (1992). Neuropsychiatric aspects of cerebral vascular disorders. In S. C. Yudofsky & R. E. Hales (Eds.), *Textbook of Neuropsychiatry (Second Edition).* Washington, DC: American Psychiatric Press.

Surawicz, F. G. (1980). Alcoholic Hallucinosis, a missed diagnosis. Differential diagnosis and management. *Canadian Journal of Psychiatry, 25,* 57–63.

Trimble, M. R. (1984). Interictal psychoses of epilepsy. *Acta Psychiatrica Scandinavica* (suppl), 313, 9–18.

Varney, N. R., Martzke, J. S., & Roberts R. J. (1987). Major depression in patients with closed head injury. *Neuropsychology, 1,* 7–9.

Wells, C. E. (1985). Organic mental disorders. In H. I. Kaplan & B. J. Sadock (Eds.), *Comprehensive Textbook of Psychiatry, 4th Ed.* Baltimore: Williams and Wilkins.

Whitehouse, P. J., Friedland, R. P., & Strauss, M. E. (1992). Neuropsychiatric aspects of degenerative dementias associated with motor dysfunction. In S. C. Yudofsky & R. E. Hales (Eds.), *Textbook of Neuropsychiatry (Second Edition).* Washington, DC: American Psychiatric Press.

Whybrow, P. C., Prange, A. J., & Treadway, C. R. (1969). Mental changes accompanying thyroid gland dysfunction. *Archives of General Psychiatry, 20,* 48–63.

Wilson, L. G. (1976). Viral encephalopathy mimicking functional psychosis. *American Journal of Psychiatry, 133,* 165–170.

Wise, M. G. & Brandt, G. T. (1992). Delirium. In S. C. Yudofsky & R. E. Hales (Eds.), *Textbook of*

Neuropsychiatry (Second Edition). Washington, DC: American Psychiatric Press.

Yudofsky, S. C. & Hales, R. E. (Eds.) (1992). *Textbook of Neuropsychiatry (Second Edition).* Washington, DC: American Psychiatric Press.

Zilboorg, G. (1941). *A History of Medical Psychology.* New York: W. W. Norton.

Zucker, D. K., Livingston, R. L., Nakra, R., & Clayton, P. J. (1981). B12 deficiency and psychiatric disorders: Case report and literature review. *Biological Psychiatry,* 16, 197–205.

Zwil, A. S., Bowring, M. A., Price, T. R. P., et al. (1990). ECT in the presence of a brain tumor: Case reports and a review of the literature. *Convulsive Therapy* 6, 299–307.

INDEX